T0313988

Kleinians

For Desmond
with gratitude and love

Kleinians

Psychoanalysis Inside Out

Janet Sayers

Polity

Copyright © Janet Sayers 2000

The right of Janet Sayers to be identified as author of this work has been asserted in accordance with the Copyright, Designs and Patents Act 1988.

First published in 2000 by Polity Press in association with Blackwell Publishers Ltd

Editorial office:
Polity Press
65 Bridge Street
Cambridge CB2 1UR, UK

Marketing and production:
Blackwell Publishers Ltd
108 Cowley Road
Oxford OX4 1JF, UK

Published in the USA by
Blackwell Publishers Inc.
350 Main Street
Malden, MA 02148, USA

All rights reserved. Except for the quotation of short passages for the purposes of criticism and review, no part of this publication may be reproduced, stored in a retrieval system, or transmitted, in any form or by any means, electronic, mechanical, photocopying, recording or otherwise, without the prior permission of the publisher.

Except in the United States of America, this book is sold subject to the condition that it shall not, by way of trade or otherwise, be lent, re-sold, hired out, or otherwise circulated without the publisher's prior consent in any form of binding or cover other than that in which it is published and without a similar condition including this condition being imposed on the subsequent purchaser.

ISBN 0-7456-2123-6
ISBN 0-7456-2124-4 (pbk)

A catalogue record for this book is available from the British Library and has been applied for from the Library of Congress.

Typeset in 10.5 on 12 pt Plantin
by Best-set Typesetter Ltd., Hong Kong
Printed in Great Britain by TJ International, Padstow, Cornwall

This book is printed on acid-free paper.

Contents

Acknowledgements

My thanks to fellow psychoanalytic psychotherapists and patients, and to students and colleagues in the Sociology Department of the University of Kent, from whom I have learnt so much over the years regarding issues dealt with in this book; to Jill Duncan, the librarian at the London Institute of Psychoanalysis; to the library of the World Health Organization in Geneva; and to the British Academy for helping fund my travel to Sydney, New South Wales, to give talks based on research for the chapters about Joan Riviere and Frances Tustin. The following have also been enormously generous in reading, commenting on and editing various drafts of *Kleinians*, and in providing biographical and other observations and details: Ann Angus, Desmond Avery, David Bell, Francesca Bion, Ronald Britton, John Buss, Sue Isaacs-Elmhirst, Stephen Frosh, Martin Golding, Vickie Hamilton, Rebecca Harkin, Andreas Heyne, Shirley Hoxter, Athol Hughes, David Ingleby, Peter Jackson, Betty Joseph, Helly Langley, Isabel Menzies Lyth, Marion Milner, Brenda Morrison, Edna O'Shaughnessy, Richard Read, Maria Rhode, Angie Rosenfeld, Lottie Rosenfeld, Lesley-Ann Sayers, Sheila Spensley, Ruth Thackeray, Shirley Toulson, Graham Tustin, Steve Uglow, Elinor Wedeles, Heinz Weiss, Roger Willoughby and Richard Wollheim. They may not agree with what I have written, but their help and support have been invaluable, for which all my thanks.

Illustrations

Introduction:
Inside Out

A revolution is happening in psychology. Once it was understood to be driven by instincts inside us. Now it is recognized to be driven by the interaction of factors operating both within and beyond us. The following chapters are about this revolution. In them I tell its story through detailing the intermingled inner and outer lives and work of its main architects in Kleinian psychoanalysis.

Psychoanalysis started, of course, with Freud. It arguably originated in Freud's self-analysis at the time of his father's death in October 1896. Certainly Freud then turned his attention to his own inner world. And this resulted in many of the examples with which he illustrated what is generally acknowledged to be his first book of psychoanalysis, namely *The Interpretation of Dreams*, published in 1900. In it Freud illustrated with his own dreams his discovery that free association to the fragments of what he called our dreams' 'manifest content' reveals them to be constructed from a ragbag of condensed and displaced memories from the previous day together with long-ago, inwardly repressed and unconscious wishes from the past.

Freud drew attention to the dynamic interplay between these aspects of our psychology. He characterized our inner world, at least its unconscious aspects, as mediated by what he called 'primary process', visual, 'pleasure principle' thinking. He contrasted it with our consciously perceived outer world which he depicted as mediated by 'secondary process', verbal, 'reality principle' thinking.

He went on to chart the development of the sexual instinct – or libido – which he initially believed to be the sole driving force of our psychology. He described this instinct as at first centring on eating, then on shitting, and finally, beginning in late infancy, on masturbating. He described this last 'psychosexual' stage of late infancy as giving rise to a phantasy[1] of getting rid of one parent to sexually enjoy the other. He famously likened this 'complex', as he called it, to the Greek myth of Oedipus killing his father and marrying his mother.

In discovering the inner, unconscious, sexual wishes and phantasies expressed in disguised form in his patients' symptoms and dreams, Freud found that his patients transferred these phantasies from the past into the present, specifically into their 'transference' relation with him. He noted that this may evoke a 'countertransference' reaction in the analyst. He recommended, however, that analysts should free themselves from any such reaction, that they should avoid premature selection from and interpretation of what their patients say and do by adopting an attitude of 'evenly-suspended attention'.

Freud arrived at these conclusions through treating women and men suffering various symptoms of what he called 'transference neuroses', which could result in hysterical or obsessional behaviour. He distinguished these disorders from what he called 'narcissistic neuroses', which he began investigating just before the First World War. These patients were characterized as being so preoccupied with their inner world that they are incapable of the outer-related transference to the psychoanalyst, which he now believed to be a precondition of psychoanalytic treatment. He included within these disorders schizophrenia and psychotic depression. He theorized the latter as due to depressives taking in, or 'introjecting', outer disappointment and hatred of those they love as though they were an inner loss. It is the depressives' resulting inwardly directed love and hate that constitutes their contradictory narcissistic self-centredness and self-loathing.

Freud wrote more about this and other contradictions following the war. He now argued that we are driven by two instincts: one seeks stimulation, the other seeks to abolish it; one seeks life, the other death. He called these instincts Eros and Thanatos. He went on to describe them as impelling the boy child to love and hate his father in rivalry with him for sexual possession of his mother. Dreading lest this be punished with castration, Freud went on, the boy identifies with his father as an inner superego figure preventing him giving way to his desire for incest. This begins a division in the child's mind, Freud claimed, between an inwardly given id and an outwardly directed ego, protected and divided against itself by the superego.

Freud announced this theory in his book *The Ego and the Id*, published in 1923. It was left to his followers to develop its implications regarding other inner–outer aspects of our psychology. First and fore-most this was done by Melanie Klein. Beginning during the First World War, she began applying Freud's insights to the analysis of very young children. The result – as Klein's analysand and student Hanna Segal, put it – is that while 'the study of the adult neurosis led Freud to discover the child in the adult; the study of children led Mrs Klein to the infant in the child'.[2] It led Klein to emphasize the ubiquity of the interacting inner and outer factors governing our psychology from earliest infancy onwards.

Many of Klein's psychoanalytic colleagues were appalled by her thus extending Freud's insights. They rejected her notion that we internalize figures from our outer world from birth. Initially, they insisted, we are driven solely by inner instinct. We do not begin to internalize the outer world in the form of phantasy figures within us until our third or fourth year of life, the age at which Freud dated the beginning of the Oedipus and castration complex and the child's internalization of the father as superego defence against it. Their insistence led to bitter wrangles in psychoanalysis in Vienna and London before and during the Second World War. But Klein's ideas survived, and with them Freud's insights were extended still further to treat schizophrenics and autistic children; our understanding of the inner–outer creative and destructive factors that shape our every-day individual, interpersonal and group psychology, both in sickness and in health, was thus enormously enhanced.

This book aims to explain how this extension, and continuing extension and expansion, of our understanding of psychology first came about. I begin with Klein. In my first chapter I argue that her account of our inner–outer psychological dynamics stemmed, at least in part, from the paradoxical mixture of loss, deprivation, rejection and intrusion she suffered in her early years. This led her to seek psy-choanalytic treatment for herself, and to begin analysing very young children, beginning with her own. I show how this in turn led her to note the centrality to mental health of recognizing and internalizing others as loved, loving and good, free from being spoilt by what she called 'paranoid-schizoid position' and 'depressive position' anxieties involving hatefully intrusive envy and expropriating greed.

I then turn to Susan Isaacs. More than anyone else, she ensured the popularization of Klein's ideas during the 1930s and 1940s through her work as a progressive school headmistress, child psy-chology journalist, head of England's first university-based child development department and leading child policy expert. In chapter 2 I explain how these achievements were perhaps driven by the unhappiness Isaacs suffered as a child, which made her want to protect others from a similar fate; she did so by familiarizing those looking after children with the phantasies they invent to bring their inner and outer worlds together.

Isaacs's analyst, Joan Riviere, explored these phantasies still further. As a young woman she had been involved in London's Bloomsbury society, now often associated with snobbery and sexual libertarianism. In chapter 3 I describe how Riviere drew on this experience to expose the dynamic interaction between our inner world and its outer feminine and masculine manifestations. In the process she exposed the fear, anger, contempt and sometimes utter desolation of the inner world, which she arguably knew first-hand from the results of her outer haughty savaging of many with whom she lived and worked.

Riviere's most moving account of this inner–outer dynamic was described in her essay 'A contribution to the analysis of the negative therapeutic reaction'. Its publication in 1936 coincided with the beginning of the major work of another Kleinian, Adrian Stokes. In the 1930s Stokes innovatively drew on his analysis by Klein of the distress he suffered following the death in the First World War of his oldest brother, Philip. He noted the value of ballet and art in giving outward mass and stability to what we experience inwardly as disturbingly fluid and fraught, as explored in chapter 4. I go on to explain how, as Stokes became happier following his second marriage, he emphasized the virtues of the visual and performing arts in so far as they repair what is damaged within us, and envelop us inwardly through what he called their 'out-thereness'.

The psychiatrist and psychoanalyst Herbert Rosenfeld, Stokes's fellow Kleinian, was more concerned to treat the ills done by this inside-out process going awry. In his later work he drew attention to the harm done to our outer lives by gangster-like figures within us. He first discovered these figures through treating women and men suffering from schizophrenia, a condition he first analysed in a woman invalided out of the Land Army during the Second World War. Rosenfeld understood schizophrenia as involving terror of being imprisoned in, or intruded into by others. In chapter 5 I argue that, in his devotion to interpreting and alleviating his patients' inner–outer fears, Rosenfeld was arguably impelled by a similar inner–outer dynamic in himself: to flee from what was going on in his immediate family to attend to others oustide.

Rosenfeld attended to the figures his patients transferred from their inner world on to him. His psychoanalyst colleague Wilfred Bion also attended to the impact on analysts of being made the outer repository of their patients projecting into them inner images, figures and fragments from within their minds. In this, as argued in chapter 6, Bion continued a tendency he recalled from when he was eight of being made the repository of his fellow pupils' unhappiness at boarding school. This was followed by his being made the repository of his fellow officers' longing for a hero in the First World War. In this sense he was something akin to the title figure of *Waiting for Godot* (written in 1952) by Samuel Beckett who was a patient of Bion's in the 1930s. Later Bion found the psychotherapy groups he began running during and after the Second World War made him into a god-like leader, responsible for everything, good and bad. Later still he found his individual patients, students and colleagues lionizing him as an omniscient deity.

In 1968 Bion moved to Los Angeles. Four years before his London-based Kleinian colleague Esther Bick had published her pioneering work, introducing infant observation to psychotherapy training – an innovation now increasingly adopted in this and other trainings across the world. In chapter 7 I seek to show how Bick arrived at this innovation through recognizing the formative impact on her own life of her experience of being mothered by her grandmother as a baby. Her grandmother's care enabled her to withstand the hardships she suffered as a child and later as a young woman when she left first Poland for Vienna, and then Vienna for London and Manchester, where she lived during the Second World War. Observing babies also alerted Bick to ways in which lack of internalizing good care as a baby, and lack of inner care and integration generally, may drive children and adults to take refuge in outer clinging to what Bick called a 'second skin'.

Frances Tustin, one of Bick's students, drew on a rather different childhood experience. Whereas Bick was separated from her mother in early infancy, Tustin remained very close to her mother into her late twenties. In chapter 8 I suggest that this closeness contributed to Tustin's pioneering understanding of anorexia and autism. The latter she described as involving fleeing recognition of separation and inner lack of integration through clinging on to outer objects and shapes. For many years Tustin argued that we all initially go through a stage of 'normal primary autism', involving intense closeness with our mothers in which we have no sense of being separate, inside or out. In this Tustin implicitly took issue with Klein's claim that, from the very start of life, the baby knows he is separate from his mother.[3]

Unlike Tustin, Hanna Segal, whose work I outline in chapter 9, has always remained absolutely faithful to Klein's major tenets. But Segal also goes beyond them in developing Klein's insights. She emphasizes the importance of facing inner separation and loss so as to forge the symbols needed to communicate with others. Segal has been especially innovative in exploring the implications of Klein's work for psychosis, literature, art and politics. Her involvement in these last three fields arguably came from her father. As for her attention to inner separation and loss, this may in part have come from her experience, aged two, of her sister dying, and from often losing her home: at the age of twelve she lost her native Poland when the family moved to Geneva; after a brief return to Warsaw she was forced by war to live first in Paris and then in London. In London she was the first to treat a schizophrenic psychoanalytically – a man whose breakdown began during his war service in India.

The exile he and Segal suffered is not, of course, universal. But we all suffer exile in the sense that we all learn early in life that we are outside, and in this sense exiled, from our mothers. We learn that our mothers are outside, independent of, and separate from us. Segal draws attention to the deleterious effect of negating our separateness from others by equating ourselves with them. *In extremis* this is expressed in psychotic equation of symbols with the people and things they symbolize.

Segal's student and colleague Ronald Britton exemplifies another aspect of this process. Drawing perhaps on his experience of being a father, and now of being a grandfather, he alerts us to ways in which our psychology is shaped by our variously recognizing our parents' sexual involvement with each other, or fleeing from it into inner illusion. Britton illustrates the point with examples from his clinical work with children and adults, and with examples from poetry, notably from Rainer Maria Rilke's *Duino Elegies*.

Britton highlights the inspiring illumination of outer experience by what Rilke called an 'angel' within us. This brings me to my conclusion, regarding the illuminating integration of inner and outer reality theorized by the Kleinians whose lives and work are the main concern of this book. It also brings me to other integrations now being furthered by Kleinian-influenced theory, not only within psychoanalysis and therapy, but also within the social sciences, humanities and politics. In looking at the precursors of these integrations I have not sought to make a comprehensive survey of Kleinianism. Indeed I have left out many very important Kleinians. But I hope that, through learning about those whose lives and work I discuss, readers will want to find out more about the revolution they and others have brought about in our understanding of the inside-out factors shaping our psychology. Now, without more ado, I begin with Klein.

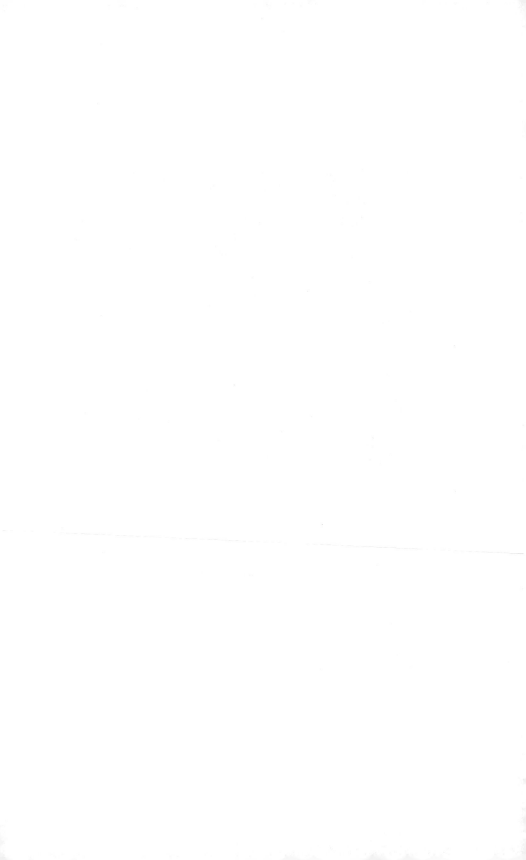

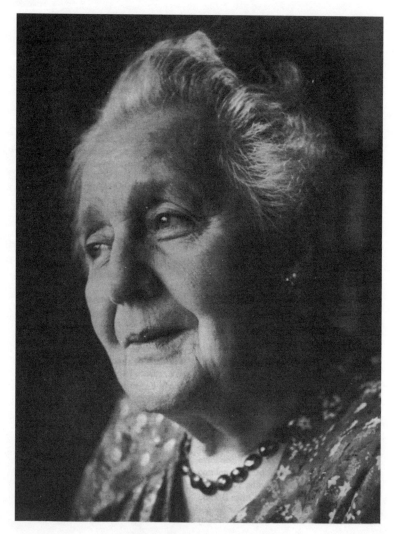

Melanie Klein, *c.*1958

1 Melanie Klein: Discovering Inner Reality

The life of Melanie Klein might not seem a very promising beginning. Her biography by Phyllis Grosskurth tells a dispiriting tale of her life as a mixture of intrusiveness, loss and rejection. Yet these very factors may well have led to what is most inspiring about Klein's work – her discoveries about our inner world, about children's phantasies of intruding into their mothers' bodies, and about the centrality in our lives of recognizing love free from 'paranoid-schizoid' and 'depressive' defences and anxieties. These terms are explained in this chapter. First, however, I discuss the intrusiveness of Klein's early mothering.

Early intrusion[1]

Melanie Klein was born in Vienna on 30 March 1882. She was the youngest of four children and seems to have been something of an afterthought. Unlike her older sisters and brother – Emilie, Emmanuel and Sidonie (who were six, five and four when she was born) – she was not breastfed by their mother, Libussa. Instead she was wetnursed. In later years she remembered feeling rejected – particularly by her father, Moriz Reizes. He had trained as a doctor and later practised as a dentist. He made no secret of his preference for Melanie's sister Emilie, who in turn ganged up with Emmanuel in teasing her. Melanie found comfort with her other sister, Sidonie, who, she later claimed, taught her to read and count, although perhaps this is unlikely given that Sidonie died, after a long illness with glandular TB, when Melanie was four.

Sidonie's death was the first of many losses. Initially Melanie was consoled by Emmanuel. He encouraged her creative writing when she was nine, and, on becoming an arts student, he introduced her to the cultural life of *fin de siècle* Vienna and to his friends, many of whom, it seems, fell in love with her. They included their second cousin, Arthur Klein, a graduate in chemical engineering from Zurich. He asked Melanie to marry him. Although she was only seventeen and already recognized that they were ill-suited, she agreed. She also knew that marrying would mean abandoning her plans to study medicine for which she had moved to a school which could prepare her for university entrance.

Perhaps Melanie was persuaded to marry Arthur by Emmanuel's high opinion of his good job prospects, her family's poverty, and the death of her father, Moriz. Her engagement was further determined by her mother, Libussa, who reacted to Moriz's death by sending her to stay with Arthur's family in Rosenberg (now called Ružomberok in today's Slovakia). Libussa thereby sought to make room for Emilie to move in with her husband, Otto, so he could take over Moriz's dental practice. She also made room by encouraging Emmanuel to stay abroad travelling. He was keen to do so in the limited time left to him due to his suffering heart disease since being ill with rheumatic fever when he was twelve.

Libussa kept Emmanuel and Melanie away. At the same time she pressed them to keep close to her emotionally by encouraging them to confide in her. Emmanuel also confided in Melanie. He plied her with complaints about his lack of money, his envy of her having so many more years to live than he did, and with tales of her fiancé's probable infidelities to her in Italy and America where Arthur was now studying. On the night of 1 December 1902, having written to Melanie complaining about the brevity of her last letter to him, Emmanuel died of heart failure in a hotel in Genoa.

Melanie was desolate. She was still grieving for Emmanuel when she married Arthur a few months later. She was just twenty-one and was disgusted by her first night's sex. During her ensuing pregnancy her mother wrote comparing her unfavourably with Emilie, and the happiness she had apparently enjoyed during her first pregnancy. Melanie, meanwhile, sought to allay her unhappiness by arranging for her late brother's writing to be published. And when her daughter Melitta was born on 19 January 1904, she threw herself into mothering.

By then relations in Vienna between Libussa and Emilie were becoming increasingly strained. Libussa reacted by intruding more into Melanie's life. She wrote complaining that Melanie had not invited her to join her and Arthur on their first holiday alone together after Melitta's birth. Then, following Melanie's depression during her next pregnancy, and after the birth of her second child Hans on 2 March 1907, Libussa moved in with the Kleins. She also seems to have taken over Melanie's place in running their home. Melanie herself later recalled enjoying having her mother living with them. But Libussa encouraged Melanie to go away, which Melanie often did. Her absences included staying in a sanatorium in Switzerland in May and June 1909. The following year Libussa moved the family to Budapest, leaving Melanie in Hermanetz, the last of a succession of small towns in Silesia to which Arthur's job had taken them, the dreariness of which had contributed to her depression.

Melanie soon joined her family. Her spirits now revived. It was then that she first became involved in psychoanalysis. She read Freud's *Interpretation of Dreams*, and about 1912 went into analysis with Sandor Ferenczi. Now it was Libussa's turn to become depressed. She became increasingly wretched and ill with cancer. Libussa's death on 6 November 1914 (only months after the birth of the Kleins' third child, Erich, on 1 July) left Melanie feeling full of guilt and regret, but even more, she later wrote, full of love for her mother and gratitude for her unstinting concern and for her serenity at the end.

Now it was Melanie's turn to become the intrusive mother. Encouraged by Ferenczi's advocacy of child analysis, she began analysing Erich. She reported her findings in a paper to the psycho-analytic congress held in Budapest in 1919. In it she described how, following a period of somewhat slow development, Erich, then aged four, asked lots of questions such as 'How is a person made?', 'What is a papa needed for?', 'What is a mamma needed for?'[2] She explained to him how the child grows inside the mother's body. Thus enlightened, he became less inhibited about investigating the world around him. He began asking more questions: about how dogs and chickens are born; about how the sun and rain are made; about God; about money, the war, and food shortages; and about the difference between wanting and getting, wishing and reality.

Meanwhile the world outside was undergoing tremendous upheaval. The end of the war and the dismantling of the Austro-Hungarian Empire was succeeded by the Bolshevik revolution in Hungary followed by a violently anti-Semitic counter-revolution. Arthur Klein – who had been invalided back from the war in 1916 – lost his job and, in the autumn of 1919, went to work in Sweden. Melanie took the children to live with his parents in Rosenberg, where she continued to analyse Erich. Following the move he was increasingly clinging. He lost interest in stories and in playing. He became increasingly silent apart from monotonously asking, 'What is the door made of?', 'What is the bed made of?', 'How is wood made?', 'How is glass made?', 'How is the chair made?', 'Where do stones, where does water come from?' and so on.[3] Melanie understood these questions to be impelled by unconscious anxiety about how he had been made – this being expressed in his also asking which plants grow from seeds – so she decided to explain human fertilization to him. It led him to recall how his playmates had told him a cock was needed for a hen to lay an egg. He became less gloomy and inhibited, and laughed when Melanie told him the story of the woman whose husband no sooner wished a sausage on the end of her nose than it grew there. He began enjoying many other stories and phantasies, including one in which two cows were walking together and one jumped on the other and rode on top of her.

But he was still bothered by the idea of babies growing inside their mothers. He wanted to see inside his mother. He wanted to see the faeces inside her as though he thought that, like faeces, babies were made from food. To this Klein responded that babies are not made from food but from 'something that papa makes and the egg that is inside mamma'. With this Erich became curious. 'I would so much like to see how a child is made inside like that',[4] he said. Then he went on to entertain lively phantasies of joining forces with his father or fighting him – phantasies in which he figured variously as a toy motor, a king or as a soldier entering his mother as though she were an electric car, a beautiful house or a garden.

He became anxious again when Klein left to go to the psychoanalytic congress of 1920 in The Hague. Here she met Karl Abraham, Freud's leading follower at that time. He invited her to settle in Berlin which, under Abraham's leadership, was then fast rivalling Vienna as a centre of psychoanalysis. First she returned to Rosenberg, where she found Erich increasingly angry. His anger was relieved, she claimed, by her continuing his analysis. For example, she analysed his saying when he urinated, 'The cow is letting down milk into the pot',[5] as a phantasy involving an unconscious image of her having a penis. He became more chatty and playful. He played, for instance, at getting under the bedclothes as though, he said, he were getting into her.

Klein concluded that addressing such phantasies is crucial to children's well-being. Otherwise they risk becoming withdrawn and inhibited, as apparently happened to her older son, Hans. Or they may lose their initial curiosity, as happened to her daughter, Melitta. Melitta, it seems, was inhibited in doing arithmetic. She could add numbers if they were the same, but not if they were different. Nor could she solve algebraic equations involving two unknowns. She was inhibited in tackling both problems, Klein wrote,[6] because they evoked ideas about sexual difference, and about Melanie's and Arthur's sexual involvement with each other, which Melitta did not want to think about. Similarly Hans was inhibited about playing games. He could not play football, for instance, because it evoked a phantasy of girls' breasts, of caressing them, and of this resulting in his being punished with castration – an anxiety exacerbated by his having undergone an operation on his penis when he was three, and by his father's punitiveness towards him on his return from the war when Hans was nine.

Hans also suffered a tic. It involved three stages: first feeling as if the hollow in his neck under the back of his head was being torn; second, feeling impelled to throw back and turn his head from side to side; and, third, feeling he had to press his chin down as far as possible. The whole movement, said Klein,[7] repeated a time before Hans was six when he shared her and his father's bedroom and wanted to be involved in their love-making. With the tic's first two movements, she said, he identified with her seeming passivity in sex, and with the last movement he identified with his father's active drilling into her.

Whether or not Hans's tic involved phantasies of intruding into her sexual intercourse with his father, and however shocking Klein's intrusiveness into her children's lives was in analysing and interpreting their phantasies in these terms, her attention to them shifted psychoanalysis from Freud's instinct-based approach to one that was more alert to children's inner images of the relations between others and themselves. But demonstrating the validity and therapeutic value of this insight depended on applying and testing it with children other than her own. Klein began to do this when, leaving Melitta in Rosenberg and Hans in a boarding school in the Tatra Mountains, she moved with Erich in January 1921 to Berlin. Here she began analysing children of members of the Berlin Psychoanalytic Society, of which she became an associate member in 1922.

Child analysis

Through analysing other people's children, Klein turned the attention of child analysis to children's transference on to the analyst of phantasies about their parents. An example was a two-year-old patient whom Klein called Rita, referred for treatment because of night terrors, animal phobias, obsessionality and depression. Initially, in analysis with Klein, Rita was too terrified to play or talk. At this Klein suggested they go outside into the garden. Here Rita became less fearful, especially after Klein explained how being alone with her in her nursery reminded her of her fear that, when she was alone in her bedroom at night, a mother-like figure might attack her. Putting this fear into words led Rita to become less fearful. She was able to return with Klein to the nursery, where her analysis continued. It then emerged that her greatest night terror was that something would come in through the window and bite her, just as she had wanted to bite and attack her mother when she was pregnant with her brother. Following his birth, this biting figure remained in her mind, stopping her playing with her doll lest she attack it.[8]

Klein treated these and other fears and inhibitions by going to Rita's home to see her. Subsequently, and to lessen children's resistance to transferring their inner phantasies about their parents on to her as their analyst, Klein began treating children away from their families in her home in the Berlin suburb of Dahlem, to which she and Arthur and their three children moved in 1923. She also provided her child patients with toys – little wooden men and women, carts, carriages, motor cars, trains, animals, bricks and houses – as well as with water, beakers, spoons, paper, scissors, pencils and paints.

From their play in analysis Klein learnt more about children's inner and outer worlds. An example was an inhibited and fearful three-year-old, Peter. His difficulties, said Klein, stemmed from witnessing his parents making love when he was eighteen months old. In his first treatment session with her, she claimed, he represented the phantasies this evoked. First he put some toy carriages and cars behind each other. Then he put them side by side. After this he knocked two toy horses together and said, 'And now they are going to sleep'. Then he buried the two horses with bricks, saying 'Now they're quite dead'. Another time he put two pencils together on a sponge and shouted at them in his father's voice. He castigated them as he had wanted to castigate his parents getting together in sex. He told them: 'You're not to go about together all the time and do piggish things'.[9]

But this gave rise to a fearful image of his father taking revenge on him. More often, however, Klein found that children are less fearful initially of their fathers than of their mothers, as was the case with a four-year-old patient, Ruth. Transferring a fearful image of her mother on to Klein, Ruth was initially so frightened of her that she had to be accompanied by her elder sister when she came to see Klein. One day she rummaged in her sister's bag and then shut it tight – 'so that nothing should fall out', she explained. She did the same with her sister's purse. Then she drew a tumbler with balls inside it and a lid on top – 'to prevent the ball from rolling out', she said. It was the same with her mother. She wanted to keep her babies safely shut up inside her mother, to stop them coming out and upsetting her as she had been upset when her younger sister was born.

Another time she played at giving dolls jugfuls of milk to drink. But when Klein put a wet sponge near one of them, Ruth insisted: 'No, she mustn't have the big sponge, that's not for children, that's for grown-ups!'. She could not bear to have what her mother had, the sponge representing her father's penis inside. Or so Klein said, maintaining that this and other aspects of Ruth's play demonstrated how much Ruth envied and could not abide what she imagined her mother had inside her – milk, penis, babies. It made her want to get into her and harm or rob her of what was inside. But this led to her imagining her mother similarly attacking her, and to her transferring this fear on to Klein.[10]

Klein argued that the phantasies involved originate in children feeling deprived by the mother of milk and faeces when they are first weaned and potty-trained. That children might indeed feel deprived of their faeces was indicated by another patient, three-year-old Trude. In analysis she pretended it was night, and that she and Klein were both asleep. Then she came over to Klein and threatened to hit her in the stomach, take out her faeces and make her poor. At this she was terrified. She hid behind the sofa, covered herself, sucked her fingers and wet herself. She thereby re-enacted, it turned out, a night-time scenario in which, when she was not quite two, she used to run into her parents' bedroom as though wanting to rob her pregnant mother of her baby. But this made her fearful lest her mother – and, by transference, Klein – similarly rob her insides. It was this, said Klein,[11] that led to the night terrors for which Trude was originally referred for treatment.

Klein presented some of these findings to the Salzburg congress held in April 1924. That month Melitta, now a medical student, married a friend of Freud's, Walter Schmideberg. Melitta's marriage was followed by her parents' divorce. Its stresses had led Melanie to go into analysis with Abraham, and to leave Arthur and move into a hotel with Erich.

That autumn, at a congress in Würzburg, Klein spoke more about children's primitive phantasies of biting and getting into their mothers, and about their phantasies of their mothers getting into them. She illustrated the point with the example of an only child, six-year-old Erna, referred for analysis because of obsessive head-banging, rocking, thumb-sucking and compulsive mastur-bating. Erna's symptoms had begun after a holiday when she was two and shared her parents' bedroom when, Erna later told her grandmother, 'Daddy got into bed with Mummy and wiggle-woggled with her'.[12]

In her analysis, it seems, Erna repeatedly acted out the phantasies to which this gave rise. Sometimes she cast Klein in the role of the mother cruelly excluding her from the oral, anal and genital pleasures she imagined her mother enjoying with her father. Oral pleasures included having Klein suck an engine with gilded lamps – 'all red and burning' – as she imagined her mother sucking her father's penis. Then, taking her mother's place, she sucked the lamps herself. She also sucked her thumb. Other times she played at 'wurling' fish with a policeman-father, while Klein had to look on as the excluded child trying to get in and take the fish from them. Still other times she pretended to dirty herself, pressed Klein to scold her, and then retaliated by vomiting up bad food, whereupon she became anxious that Klein might similarly attack her. She talked, for instance, of a flea, all 'black and yellow mixed', like a piece of food or shit, coming out of Klein's body and forcing itself into her.

Through having these phantasies interpreted and explained, Klein claimed, Erna began to distinguish more clearly between her inner image of her mother as fearful and attacking and what her mother actually was outside. As a result, Klein added, Erna's image of her mother became less harsh and frightening; her play became more warmly maternal and tender as she felt less driven by her feelings not only of deprivation but of envy of her mother to ward off these feelings with the obsessional symptoms which had brought her into treatment.

Whatever the success of Erna's analysis in allaying these symptoms, her primitive oral and anal talk – including talk of making her parents into 'mincemeat' and 'eye-salad' – was hardly the stuff that would endear Klein to her Berlin colleagues. They denounced her work as embarrassing and ridiculous. They said she was 'feeble-minded about theory'.[13] Psychoanalysts in Vienna were similarly critical when Klein spoke to them about her work in December 1924. Members of the British Psycho-Analytical Society, however, proved more sympathetic to Klein's ideas when James Strachey gave them an account of her Vienna talk the next month, having learnt about its contents from his wife Alix (who, like Klein, was also in analysis with Abraham in Berlin).

This led to Klein being invited to give talks about her work in London in July 1925. Her return afterwards to Berlin, however, was bleak. An affair she had begun that spring ended. And that Christmas Abraham suddenly died, leaving her nobody to defend her against her detractors in Berlin. She therefore gladly accepted an invitation she now received from Ernest Jones, the founding President of the British Psycho-Analytical Society, to analyse his children. In September 1926 she moved to London. Here she lived first in a flat in the Temple and then in a maisonette near the Institute of Psycho Analysis (then housed in Gloucester Place). After Erich arrived at the end of the year she settled in Notting Hill, from where he went to school at St Paul's.

Meanwhile Freud's psychoanalyst daughter, Anna, gave lectures in Vienna attacking Klein's method of child analysis. Her lectures were published in 1927.[14] The same year, in a symposium held in London on 4 and 18 May, Klein replied.[15] She rejected Anna Freud's claim that children are too closely involved with their parents to entertain phantasies about them. She illustrated the gap between children's inner phantasies about their parents and their outer reality with the example of a four-year-old patient, Gerald.

Outwardly, said Klein, Gerald had never been punished or threatened by his parents. Inwardly, however, he imagined them eating him, cutting him to pieces and castrating him – phantasies he transferred on to Klein in analysis in which he variously imagined her as an idealized fairy godmother or as a wicked witch. It is these figures in children's minds and their transposition into others outside, Klein claimed, that inhibit their play. Freeing children from inhibition accordingly depends on exposing and reducing the harshness of these figures rather than strengthening them, as Anna Freud advocated, in seeking to reinforce the child's superego.

Klein went on to summarize the findings of her approach in a talk to the congress held in Innsbruck in September 1927. Here she maintained that children's first phantasies are about their mothers.[16] She therefore described children's initial development as constituted by a woman-centred 'femininity phase'. Subsequently, she said, the sexes diverge. Boys fend off fear of the mother as a terrifying inner figure with the reassurance that, whatever attacks they dread from her, their penis remains intact. Girls, by contrast, having no such outward reassurance because their sexual organs are inside, are less able to allay their phantasies about what they or their mothers might have done to their sexuality.

Soon after speaking about these issues in Innsbruck Klein was elected to full membership of the British Psycho-Analytical Society. In May 1929 she spoke to the society about Maurice Ravel's opera *L'enfant et les sortilèges*, with a libretto by Colette. It begins with a little boy not wanting to do his homework. He would much rather go to the park, pull the cat's tail and scold everyone, particularly his mother. When she comes in and asks if he has finished, he puts his tongue out at her, whereupon she punishes him saying, 'You shall have dry bread and no sugar in your tea'.[17] At this he flies into a rage, attacks the tea things, the pets, the fire and the pendulum inside a grandfather clock – just as the Oedipal child, said Klein, seeks to attack his father inside his mother. But then everything comes alive. A wild rumpus starts – not unlike that depicted in Maurice Sendak's children's book *Where the Wild Things Are*. The little boy tries to find refuge in the park. But he is attacked there too. Animals fight and bite him, just as, Klein said, he wanted to attack his mother. But then a squirrel falls to the ground beside him. He picks it up and binds its injured paw. With this his world becomes more friendly. The once fearsome figures – the animals representing his inner world – appreciate his kindness and he is restored to his mother.

In the same talk Klein used another example, that of Ruth Kjär, a Scandinavian artist. Beautiful, rich and independent, Kjär also suffered occasional bouts of depression in which she felt unbearably empty inside. This was matched by emptiness outside, particularly by the blankness of a wall from which her artist brother-in-law had taken down one of his paintings. It made Kjär feel emptier than ever. It impelled her to fill the space. She herself started painting – pictures of a black woman, of her sister and of an old woman all wrinkled and worn. They culminated in a portrait of her mother – magnificent, imperious and challenging.

By then, in 1928, Klein had been joined by her daughter Melitta in London. From early May 1930 Melitta is also recorded as regularly attending meetings of the British Psycho-Analytical Society. In early July 1930 the society officially recognized the discipline of child analysis which Klein had done so much to develop. It agreed rules for its members' child psychoanalysis training. Klein's account of her analysis of a four-year-old, Dick, was also published in 1930.[18] She described him as schizophrenic; nowadays he would probably be diagnosed as autistic.

She describes how, as a baby, Dick was so apathetic in feeding and sucking that he nearly died of starvation. He was also seemingly starved of affection by his mother and wetnurse. But, with the help of another nurse and his grandmother, he survived. Gradually he was toilet-trained and, with time, he also learnt a few words. By the age of four, however, he still refused to eat anything but pap. Eating or engaging with anything caused him too much anxiety. It evoked fears of terrifyingly destructive intrusion into others, and of their retaliatory intrusion into him against which he defended himself by shutting himself off from all involvement with others, and from all play, talk and curiosity about the world around him.

He was interested in nothing but trains and stations, doors and rooms. They represented his mother's body which he both wanted and was terrified of getting into. As evidence Klein cited his response to her talking to him in these terms after he began his first session with her by running aimlessly around the room. Seeking to engage him she took up two trains. She called one 'Daddy' and the other 'Dick'. At this he took up the 'Dick' train and rolled it to the window, saying 'Station'. Klein commented, 'The station is Mummy: Dick is going into Mummy'. At this he ran into the dark space between the inner and outer doors of her room. This sequence recurred in ensuing sessions. He became increasingly involved. He also became more concerned about what others felt inside. One day, for instance, he scratched a toy coal-cart, threw it into a drawer and covered it with the other toys. Then, putting the coal-cart and the drawer's other contents into Klein's lap, he said sadly, 'Poor Mrs Klein'.[19]

In 1931 Klein took on her first trainee analysand, a Canadian, Clifford Scott. Soon after that, she took on another trainee, an American, David Slight. She also supervised both men's first child analysis cases. In 1932 her first book, *The Psycho-Analysis of Children*, was published. It was greeted with enthusiasm by fellow members of the British Psycho-Analytical Society. Soon, however, enthusiasm turned to bitter disagreement following talks she now gave about depression.

Inner depression

Like Freud (see p. 2 above), Klein related depression to loss. She herself suffered a number of losses during the 1930s. She lost the friendship of her daughter, who, after her election to membership of the British Psycho-Analytical Society in April 1933, became increasingly hostile to her mother both in relation to the society and beyond it. She vehemently complained of Klein's intrusion into her life professionally and personally. To the loss of her daughter's affection was added the loss of her son Hans, who died in April 1934 in a climbing accident in the Tatra Mountains.

Hans's death left Klein utterly miserable. Prevented by grief from attending his funeral and psychoanalytic meetings in London, she devoted herself instead to working on a talk about depression for that summer's Lucerne congress.[20] In it she put forward for the first time her theory that our psychology is constituted from the very start of life – even before weaning and toilet-training begin – by love and hate of others, and by our imagining them as loved and hated figures within us. The baby, she wrote, initially takes in his mother both as good and loved, and as bad and hated. On the other hand, he also wants to get in and scoop out, devour and destroy everything inside her.

To the extent that the baby nevertheless increasingly experiences his mother as intact and whole, and as loved and good, both inside and out, he feels more able to countenance also experiencing her as bad and hated. He no longer feels so driven to divide one image from the other. But this gives rise to fear that, in attacking the mother he hates, he might have lost the mother he loves. For he now realizes the two mothers are one and the same. He fears losing her. He also feels guilt and concern that his hatred has damaged or even killed her. It impels him to try to put the damage right – to revive, repair and restore her. Or, feeling overwhelmed by the work involved, babies, children and adults defend against it with self-preoccupied manic excitement, hypochondria and persecutory fears for themselves. Klein called this constellation of fears and defences the 'depressive position' and added that we may take flight from its inner reality into outer-directed hyperactivity and omnipotent control of others, inside and out.

An example, she wrote, was a man who came for analysis suffering severe depressive, paranoid and hypochondriacal anxieties. In the course of his analysis he dreamt he was travelling with his parents in an open-topped railway carriage. He felt free as air. He felt he was 'managing the whole thing', including looking after his parents who were much older and more needy in his dream than they were in real life. He dreamt they were lying end to end in adjoining beds, and that he was trying with difficulty to keep them warm. Then he dreamt that he pissed, while they watched, into a basin, in the middle of which was a cylindrical object that he felt he must be careful not to piss into. He felt his penis was very large. He did not want his father to see it lest it make him feel too small by comparison. He also felt he was pissing for his father to save him the bother of getting up to piss for himself.

In free associating to his dream, Klein's patient said the cylindrical object reminded him of a gas-mantle and of the lights in his grandmother's house. It made him sad. It reminded him of poor and dilapidated houses with nothing alive in them but a low-burning light. Klein reminded him that in his dream he had been anxious to avoid urinating into the cylindrical object lest, as it were, his urine put out the light. This led him to dream the next night that he heard something frizzling in an oven. He thought it was brown, probably a kidney in a pan. The sound was like a tiny voice, as though something alive were being fried. Before telling Klein this dream he complained of the way she had lit her cigarette so carelessly that a bit of the match broke off and flew towards him. He also complained that he did not want to talk because he was so bunged up with a cold.

Putting all this together, Klein said his first dream indicated his concern to look after his parents, and his depressive anxiety lest he make the light or life in them go out. But he also defended against this anxiety by manically controlling and doing everything for his parents, and by retreating, in his second dream and its precursors, into feeling persecuted with frizzling and his cold inside, and externally with Klein's carelessness in lighting her cigarette.

Writing more generally, she argued that weaning is the first major loss, giving rise to a constellation of manically controlling and self-preoccupied persecutory fears and defences against depressive concern for others. Weaning conditions the baby's already internalized image and phantasies about his parents. It triggers what Klein now called the 'infantile depressive position'. She concluded from its occurrence in both children and adults, including the man in the above example, that this position is central in forming our psychology.

By now she was insisting that children have inner images and phantasies about their parents from birth. In this she implicitly disagreed with Freud's claim that we first form inner images and phantasies about our parents – as superego figures, as he called them – in resolving Oedipal conflict between sex and aggression in late infancy. To resolve this disagreement a series of exchange lectures between Klein's and Freud's supporters was held in London and Vienna in 1936. But disagreement continued. It became even more heated in 1938, following the arrival in London of Freud and his daughter, Anna, from Nazi-invaded Vienna.

Undeterred by the Freuds' arrival Klein continued to reiterate her claims regarding the infantile depressive position. She spoke further about it in a talk to the Paris congress of 1938. Reiterating her Lucerne talk of 1934, she argued that outward loss or death of those we love elicits fear of also losing them as loved figures within us. Their loss returns us to the depressive position we experienced in infancy on being weaned and toilet-trained. It also reactivates this position's associated defences, including phantasies of all-powerful triumph, denial and idealization.

Klein illustrated the point by recounting, as though it were the experience of one of her patients, her reaction to Hans's death. At first she idealized him. She kept everything she felt was good of his and threw out everything she felt was bad. She also dreamt she had not lost him, that it was not him but her brother – her mother's son

– who had died. She felt hostile to both her mother and brother in her dream, in which she also felt she controlled and triumphed over them. In a subsequent dream she imagined she was flying with Hans, that he then disappeared and drowned, but she survived; the same feelings were aroused.

This dream of triumphing over her son was followed by friendlier images. She took comfort in looking at pleasantly situated houses in the country. She thought she would like to have one for herself. She began to trust in there being good and loved things and people outside. As a result she felt less driven to control her inner world. Appreciating and taking in what she felt was good and loved outside, she felt less driven to deny Hans's death, more able to acknowledge it. With this her grief at his loss came out in full force. She took comfort in experiencing figures in her inner world as also, in a sense, grieving and crying for her. At times, however, she still retreated from recognizing Hans's loss. This included retreating from depressive anxiety and concern about his being gone to self-preoccupied feelings of being persecuted, of being overwhelmed by people in the street, of anxiety at houses seeming alien and strange, and at the thought that the sunshine was false and artificial. But her home felt secure. With time she increasingly came to experience her mother and others – previously lost to her as good figures through her denying, controlling and triumphing over them inside – as alive, loving, loved and good.

In her talk in Paris in 1938 Klein further illustrated this process of recovery with the example of how one of her patients had reacted to his mother's death. The night before she died he dreamt he was with her and that a dangerous bull was between them; he fled, leaving his mother unprotected. It reminded him of shooting buffalo to eat and of buffalo being an endangered species, needing protection. The next session he arrived hating Klein. Unconsciously he equated her with his dream image of his mother mixed up with his father as a bull. Only when Klein noted this image's counterpart – his remembering that buffalo need protection from extinction – did he tell her that his mother had died. He went on to say how sick he felt at the news. With this he gradually became more confident of feeling concerned about the protection and well-being of others, more able to acknowledge his loss of and love and longing for his 'dear old parents', as he called them. He less often saw them as the attacking and attacked figures that had previously thwarted his relations both with them and with others.[21]

In arguing that the loss and death of those we love revive anxieties and defences first experienced in the depressive position of earliest infancy, Klein reiterated the claim she had made in 1934 that this position centrally determines our subsequent psychology. After her talk of 1938 she emphasized that, far from being primary, the Oedipus complex is secondary to the depressive position, and that it is only when we have worked through this position's anxieties and defences that we feel sufficiently secure to face the conflicts of the Oedipus complex. Klein illustrated this claim with the examples of Rita (see pp. 13–14 above) and a ten-year-old boy, Richard,[22] whom she began treating at the end of April 1941 in Pitlochry in Scotland, where she had been invited by the parents of her 'schizophrenic' patient Dick to take refuge with them from the war.

Richard's ills on beginning analysis included being so fearful of other people that he had been unable to go to school since he was eight. Now he was also fearful of the war, in which his house had been bombed. Klein interpreted to him his fears and defences against them in terms of her theory of the depressive position. As a result, she claimed, he became calmer and more trusting and hopeful of others and of her. He experienced the room in which they met as cosier. He drew pictures in which his image of his mother became friendlier. He began recalling good early memories. And he sought to keep Klein as a good figure in his mind, or so Klein wrote, by having her help him tie his shoelaces, by thinking of becoming an analyst like her and by taking a photograph of her.

He thereby became more confident, maintained Klein, of having enough good figures inside to enable him to withstand and restore any damage done to himself or others by Oedipal conflict with them. He could therefore allow this conflict to come out in full force: he openly competed with the confectioner from whom he saw Klein getting her cigarettes; he willed the ironmonger to stop his loud talk intruding from across the street into the room where he and Klein met; he worried about a frail old professor in a German film; he asked Klein about her husband. He was also open about feeling sensitive lest, compared with these men, he seem too small and boy-like to her: he acknowledged hating the tobacconist for humiliating him in front of her by sending him to the back of the queue, the bus conductress for shouting, 'Half fares stand up', and his mother for thinking he was too weak to go swimming.

As he increasingly took into himself his relation with Klein as being good and helpful, he became less full of hate, resentment and anxiety in relation to others. He felt more able to return to school and to face the ending of his treatment with Klein. He regretted it finishing. But he felt hopeful of coping with its loss, both through touching Klein several times during their last meeting and through feeling that his treatment had made her securely lodged as a good and helpful figure within him.

For Klein the ending of his analysis was followed by what are now known as the British Psycho-Analytical Society's Controversial Discussions, which began in 1943. Conflict between Klein's supporters and her detractors nearly tore the society apart. It was saved, however, towards the end of the war by its members agreeing to disagree through forming three groups. One followed Anna Freud, another Melanie Klein, leaving a third independent. This arrangement ensured not only the future of Klein's work, but the development of her final work, which is regarded by many as her most important contribution to psychoanalysis: her theory of what she called 'projective identification' and of the disrupting effects of envy on love.

Projective identification, envy and love

Klein first formulated her theory of projective identification in answer to an essay by the Edinburgh psychoanalyst W. R. D. Fairbairn, published in 1944, about what he believed to be a normally occurring 'schizoid position' in early infancy;[23] he claimed that the baby manages frustration by imagining his mother as a divided – exciting and tantalizing – figure within him. By contrast Klein maintained in December 1946 in a talk to the British Psycho-Analytical Society that, whatever the frustrations babies suffer, they inevitably divide their mothers as both loved and hated: experiencing the mother as hated and hateful – and therefore as persecuting – exacerbates the baby's fear from birth of fragmenting. Against these fears, she added, the baby defends himself with further fragmentation and splitting of hate from love, bad from good. This includes fragmenting and getting rid of bad figures within. It also includes idealizing the mother to protect and preserve her as loved and good, free from all contaminating and damaging contact with what is hated and bad. The baby also idealizes his mother, according to Klein, as a result of his desire for unlimited gratification impelling him to picture her as an 'inexhaustible and always bountiful breast'.[24]

Idealization and splitting, together with fragmentation and persecution, constitute what Klein now called the 'paranoid-schizoid position'. It is succeeded and offset, she went on, by our experiencing and taking our mothers and others into our minds as loved and good. This becomes an integrative force for bringing together love and hate, good and bad. It enables us to progress from paranoid-schizoid self-preoccupation to depressive position concern for others. One position flows into and alternates with the other.

The first (paranoid-schizoid) position, said Klein, includes identifying with others through exporting into them loved and hated figures from inside us. In describing this process she launched her theory of what she called 'projective identification', involving not so much projecting instincts from within us on to others, as Freud had described, but projecting and identifying with others on the basis of putting into them loved and hated figures from within us. An example, she said, was a schizophrenic patient who projected all good figures from within herself into Greta Garbo, who thereby came to stand for her. In an essay of 1955 she cited another example, which occurs in the then recently translated novel *If I Were You* (1947), by the Paris-based American Julian Green.[25] In the novel the central character, Fabian, escapes his life as a petty official, made dreary by lack of love, by making a pact with the devil; this enables him to get into and take over the lives of others and thus to enjoy the goodness he imagines and envies in them.

Envy was the subject of Klein's last major work. In 1946 she had written that paranoid-schizoid fragmentation and disintegration are counteracted by acknowledging and taking in the mother and others as loved and good figures within us. Nearly a decade later, at the international congress of psychoanalysis held in Geneva in 1955, she gave a talk, later expanded into her book *Envy and Gratitude* (1957), in which she drew attention to ways in which this process of internalizing what is loved and good may be disrupted. She noted that it may be disrupted by phantasies of greedily expropriating and emptying, and of enviously getting into and spoiling what we love and find good in others. Or we idealize them, thus mobilizing our envy still further.

She went on to highlight envy's intrusive, biting character by quoting Edmund Spenser's *Faerie Queen* (1596), in which envy is likened to a hungry wolf:

> He hated all good workes and vertuous deeds . . .
> And eke the verse of famous Poets witt
> He does backebite, and spightfull poison spues
> From leprous mouth on all that ever writt.[26]

She also illustrated envious destruction of what is loved and good in others with clinical examples. They included a woman patient who rubbished Klein in her mind by dreaming of her as an apathetic, contemptible and useless cow, looking down on her from a magic carpet. Meanwhile Klein, as the cow, munched an endless strip of blanket, as though eating her words as woolly and worthless. Klein explained to the patient the way she thus enviously spoilt the words and understanding she wanted from Klein. As a result she was gradually able to take in their relationship as good, integrating and helpful.

Klein spoke more about envy in May 1959 to a group of sociologists.[27] She also spoke about envy in her last psychoanalytic congress talk in Copenhagen that summer, in which she dwelt on loneliness. She said it involved longing for the love and understanding we first experience with our mothers. She also said loneliness involves longing to regain our mothers and other figures we have lost through attributing and putting our images of them into others. Or we lose them through envy and greed. She gave the example of a patient who sought to counteract his loneliness with enjoyment of the countryside, only to find it ruined by childhood memories of greedily robbing birds' nests and enviously damaging hedges. What he most wanted was to grow things.

Klein concluded this talk by stating that dispelling loneliness depends on overcoming envy and greed and other paranoid-schizoid and depressive obstacles to experiencing goodness and love. Once we feel grateful for our mothers and other figures, we may then arrive at old age able to enjoy our own youth in that of others. She herself was now seventy-seven. The next summer she became ill on holiday in Switzerland and was brought back to London by her student and colleague Esther Bick. Here, after an operation for cancer, she returned home. But, obstinately determined to get up, she fell, broke her hip, and soon after died, on 22 September 1960. Her obstinacy might have contributed to her death. But it also contributed to her work enduring, as did its development by Susan Isaacs, to whom I now turn.

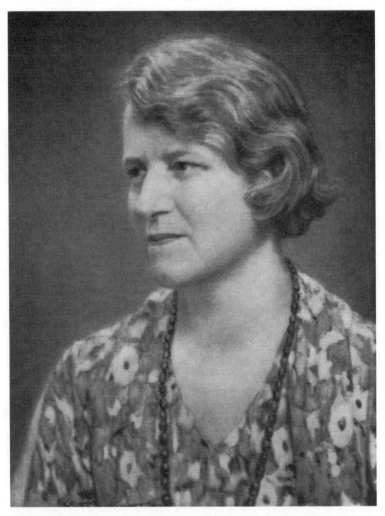

Susan Isaacs, photographed from a miniature painted in 1935 by her brother, Enoch Fairhurst

2 Susan Isaacs: Children's Phantasies

Susan Isaacs helped Klein's work to endure through the support she gave it in her contribution to the British Psycho-Analytical Society's wartime discussions. Even more important, however, was her skill as a psychologist, teacher, researcher and writer in discovering and conveying the ubiquity and early appearance of phantasy in mediating and integrating children's inner and outer worlds. In this she was driven by her concern to enable parents and others better to understand and protect children from the unhappiness she suffered as a child.

Unhappy childhood[1]

Born Susan Sutherland Fairhurst on 24 May 1885 in Bromley Cross, near Bolton in Lancashire, Susan was the ninth child of Miriam and William Fairhurst. She was weaned suddenly when her brother William became ill with pneumonia. He died, and this freed Miriam to give Susan more of her attention. But with the birth of another child, Alice, when Susan was four, she again lost Miriam's attention. Miriam became ill, and died two years later. Susan's unhappiness at her mother's death was compounded by Miriam having accused her shortly beforehand of lying in suggesting that her father was having an affair with the nurse. But it was true. Soon after Miriam's death William married the nurse.

By then, already established as a Methodist lay preacher and journalist, William had become editor of the *Bolton Journal and Guardian*. This enabled the family to move to a large house, Monksfield, on the outskirts of Bolton. But Susan was very unhappy and, still aged only six, she ran away to the house of a family friend who had several times playfully suggested they marry. He welcomed her, took her in, and sent a note to her family telling them what had happened. They replied by sending a parcel saying, if she was going to marry, she would need clothes. Opening it, however, she discovered it was stuffed with newspaper. It left her feeling utterly mocked and humiliated. It was this, she later wrote, that first launched her on her career of seeking to enable others to understand children better.

She and Alice found refuge, in the council infant school, from what one commentator called 'the tragedy' of their childhood home.[2] But the school, like home, was full of constraints and inadequacies against which Susan soon rebelled. When she was twelve she went to Bolton's recently opened secondary school. Here too she was unhappy and suffered the humiliation of being teased by the boys for being kept in short dresses by her stepmother. She also suffered her father's authoritarianism, which included punishing his children for even such minor offences as grammatical errors. Now he punished Susan by withdrawing her, aged fourteen, from school. Through her brother Enoch, she had become interested in agnosticism, to which William responded by saying 'if education makes women Godless, they are better without it'.[3]

Susan wrote of this period of her life as though it were that of a patient. It was:

> characterised by obstinacy, noisiness, insubordination, seeking after boys, occasional stealing. At seven years she ate chalk (just as some younger children insist on drinking their bath water). She used in school to blow her nose very loudly in order to annoy a woman teacher whom she much admired and loved. In early adolescence she became an intellectual rebel against everything her father believed in and had frequent feelings of utter despair, with strongly marked suicidal tendencies.[4]

She also felt miserable and guilty because it was her brother's early death that had secured for her her mother's attention as a baby. And she worried lest her jealousy of her younger sister, Alice, had contributed to Miriam's subsequent illness and death, and to the family being so 'disorderly and unhappy'.[5]

Whether or not Susan's childhood unhappiness contributed to her rebellion as a teenager, her father withdrawing her from school was followed by her working briefly as an apprentice photographer. She also helped keep house with her 'mother-sister' Bessie,[6] read a great deal, played the piano, supported the suffragette leaders Mrs

Pankhurst and Mrs Despard, refused to wear corsets, declared herself a socialist and joined the Fabian Society. When she was sixteen, she persuaded Alice to join her in giving up butter so as to send the money thus saved to support the striking cotton-mill workers. She also earned money teaching a delicate boy at home, spent a year as a nursery governess with an English family in Morocco and taught in a small private school in Bolton.

Meanwhile Miriam and Alice went to teacher training college. Eventually she persuaded her father to let her go to college as well. He agreed grudgingly, saying young children were, after all, 'the province of women'.[7] She joined a course for infant school teachers at Manchester University run by Grace Owen, an advocate of the progressive learning-by-doing ideas of Friedrich Froebel and John Dewey. Impressed by Susan's 'quite unusual intelligence',[8] Owen persuaded the professor of education, Findlay, to encourage Susan to take a degree. He did so and used his influence to persuade her father to agree. Her cousin William Sutherland coached her in the German she needed for the university entrance exam. He was also perhaps her first boyfriend. Certainly he and Susan made enquiries about cousins marrying. And he was evidently very impressed by the intelligence and hard work she put into securing a place at the university where, among many other activities, she became a founder member of the university's Socialist Federation.

Susan's father died within a year of her becoming an undergraduate. In the absence of his leaving a will his estate was divided between his widow and daughters, enabling Susan to repay her grant and thus free herself from having to become a teacher on graduating. Instead, on finishing in 1912 with a first-class degree in philosophy, she went to Newnham, Cambridge, to do research with Charles Myers, to whom one of her Manchester professors, Tom Pear, had recommended her. F. W. H. Myers was one of the first, through the Society for Psychical Research, to introduce to English readers the essay on hysteria by Josef Breuer and Sigmund Freud, published in 1893.[9] But Charles Myers was no enthusiast for psychoanalysis. He persuaded Susan to do research on children's spelling difficulties and, after completing her MA on the subject, during which time she lived in Newnham, she returned north. Here from 1913 to 1914 she lectured in infant school education at Darlington Training College, and from 1914 to 1915 taught logic at Manchester University.

In 1914 she married one of her former Manchester University teachers, the botanist William Brierley. The following year he was appointed a researcher into plant diseases at Kew Gardens in London, and the couple moved to a top-floor flat overlooking Richmond Park. Susan now got work teaching psychology for London

County Council, London University and the Workers' Educational Association (WEA). She also wrote up her MA research and began writing her first book, *An Introduction to Psychology*.[10] In the latter she emphasized the biological roots of psychology. But she was also interested in psychoanalysis. In 1921 she began a long analysis with J. C. Flügel, a close friend from Oxford of the psychologist Cyril Burt, with whom Flügel now worked at University College London (UCL). Here, following the First World War, Flügel had become the first person to teach psychoanalysis in an English university. He was also secretary of the International Psycho-Analytical Association.

Susan too combined teaching and administration. From 1919 to 1921 she was Honorary Secretary of the Education Section of the British Psychological Society (BPS) and served on the editorial board of its *Journal of Educational Psychology*. In 1921 she became an assistant editor on the *British Journal of Psychology*. Other responsibilities included serving, from 1921 to 1929, as a member of the Council of the National Institute of Industrial Psychology (NIIP, about which she also wrote),[11] and from 1923 to 1931, on the NIIP's advisory committee on vocational guidance. (Other NIIP members included Myers and – until 1927 – Marion Milner who, like Susan, also became a psychoanalyst.)

Meanwhile Susan had become involved with one of her WEA students, Nathan Isaacs. He was ten years her junior and from a Russian Jewish family which had fled from Warsaw to Basel and settled in England when he was twelve. On leaving school at fourteen he had become a junior clerk to a button merchant, and then gone into business in metals. He was keenly interested in philosophy and psychology; after becoming dissatisfied with the Aristotelian Society's version of 'mental philosophy', he pursued the subject through Susan's WEA class, to which he was introduced by an economist friend, Lionel (later Lord) Robbins. Soon, it seems, his enthusiasm for Susan led him to ply her with endless questions and a ninety-five-page essay.[12] At first Susan was reserved about these attentions. She went abroad and had a brief analysis with Otto Rank. Finally she eloped with Nathan to Austria, and got a divorce from William. (William went on to become Professor of Botany at Reading University and, after retiring, settled in the Lake District with his second wife, Marjorie, who became a psychoanalyst.)

Susan and Nathan got married in 1922 and settled in a flat in 53 Hunter Street, Bloomsbury. Because of the scandal of her getting involved with Nathan while still married to William, the WEA had stopped employing her. Instead she decided to devote herself to children. She herself never had any: neither William nor Nathan wanted them; and by the time she got over her fear of childbearing (given her mother's illness and death after her sister's birth) it was too late. Determined nevertheless to work with children, she decided to do so by becoming a medically qualified psychoanalyst. She took the necessary preliminary exams, but, having burdened Nathan with the cost of their Bloomsbury home, she was loath to burden him further with the cost of her medical training. So she abandoned it and instead trained as a non-medical lay analyst, becoming an associate member of the British Psycho-Analytical Society on 13 October 1921 and a full member on 3 October 1923.

In 1923 her first article about psychoanalysis was published. It was on sexual inequality, the overcoming of which, she argued, depends on addressing children's phantasies about the differences between the sexes. She illustrated the point with an example, perhaps taken from her own childhood, of a four-and-a-half-year-old girl who persuaded her older brother to cut off her hair, and proclaimed herself to be a boy, and then swallowed his whistle, saying 'I didn't like the noise, so I hid it in myself'.[13] In this she arguably acted on the phantasy of taking into herself what she felt stood for her brother's privileges as a boy. Having recounted this phantasy, Isaacs went on to recount many more children's phantasies following work she now took up as the headmistress of a progressive school.

Headmistress

On 22 March 1924 a full-page advertisement appeared in the *New Statesman*, announcing:

> WANTED – an Educated Young Woman with honours degree – prefer-ably first class – or the equivalent, to conduct education of a small group of children aged $2\frac{1}{2}$ –7, as a piece of scientific work and research . . . someone . . . who has hitherto considered themselves too good for teaching and who has probably already engaged in another occupa-tion. . . . Preference will be given to those who do not hold any form of religious belief.[14]

The advertisement was an expanded version of one that had also appeared in *Nature*, in the *British Journal of Psychology* and in an earlier issue of the *New Statesman*, 1 March 1924. The advertiser turned out to be a Mr Geoffrey Pyke, an investor on the London Stock Exchange, who lived near the Isaacses in a flat in Gordon Square previously occupied by the economist John Maynard Keynes.[15]

Like Susan, Geoff Pyke had had an unhappy childhood. His father, a Jewish lawyer, died when Geoff was five. Geoff was then sent to Wellington, where his mother insisted he observe the habits and adopt the dress of the orthodox Jew. There were no other Jews there, and his fellow pupils – mostly sons of army officers – mercilessly instituted 'Jew Hunts' against him. After a couple of years he left and was educated at home before going to Pembroke College, Cambridge, where he studied law. But he never finished his degree and instead, having persuaded the *News Chronicle* to take him on as a war correspondent, he went to Berlin, where he was almost immediately captured and imprisoned near Charlottenburg, in Ruhleben, from where he ensured widespread coverage of his escape.

But the miseries he suffered in prison, he later maintained, were nothing compared with those he suffered at Wellington. Determined that his children should not suffer similarly, he prepared himself for fatherhood – when his wife, Margaret, became pregnant with their first child, David – by going into analysis with James Glover, who was then practising in Wimpole Street. In 1923, when David was three, Geoff asked an American economist friend at Cambridge, Philip Sargant Florence, to send one of his sons to live with them to keep David company. Not unreasonably Florence refused, at which Geoff decided to found a school at which David would be assured of having company. With grand plans for it to become a research institute, revolutionizing children's education in freeing them to pursue whatever interests they liked,[16] he decided that the most suitable setting for the project would be the Malting House, Cambridge, which he had begun renting that year for his family.

Nathan Isaacs was intrigued by Pyke's advertisement in the *New Statesman*. Susan was more cautious. She suspected the advert was the work of a crank. But Nathan – together with Glover and Pyke, who visited the Isaacess in their Hunter Street flat – persuaded Susan to take on the post and she agreed, provided she was given sole charge of running the school. It opened on 6 October 1924 with ten two- to four-year-old boys. Soon it expanded to include a few girls. Some of the children boarded in nearby St Chad's, in Grange Road, where they were looked after by a Miss Mary Ogilvie.[17] Pupils included Sue Foss (who went on to become the Kleinian analyst Sue Isaacs-Elmhirst), G. E. Moore's sons (Nicholas and Tim who, at two and a half, was the youngest when the school started), Lord Rutherford's grandson, Lord Adrian's daughter, the Florences' younger son Tony, and, of course, the Pykes' son, David.

Recalling Susan at the time, the psychoanalyst John Rickman (who had worked with W. R. H. Rivers as a psychiatrist in Cambridge's mental hospital, Fulbourn)[18] described her as sturdy, chubby, rather short, challenging, friendly, dumbfounding but forebearing and also 'rather cold'. The psychoanalyst James Strachey was much more critical. He dismissed her as 'conceited beyond words'.[19] As for her

school – dubbed by some a 'pre-genital brothel'[20] – Strachey wrote
of its pupils:

> All that appears to happen is that they're allowed to do whatever they
> like. But as all they like doing is kicking one another, Mrs Isaacs is
> obliged to intervene in a sweetly reasonable voice: 'Timmy, please do
> not insert that stick in Stanley's eye'. There is one particular boy (age
> 5) who domineers, and bullies the whole set. His chief enjoyment is
> spitting. He spat one morning onto Mrs Isaacs's face. So she says: 'I
> shall not play with you Philip' – for Philip is typically his name – 'unless
> you have wiped my face.' As Philip didn't want Mrs Isaacs to play with
> him, that lady had to go about the whole morning with the crachat
> upon her. Immediately Tony appeared Philip spat at him, and in
> general cowed and terrified him as had never happened to him
> before.[21]

Isaacs herself also noted what her pupils said and did. She kept
a diary of their biological interests and phantasies, including the
following observation of their playing while dissecting mice:

> 20.7.26 Christopher, Dan, and Priscilla dissected one each. . . . While
> dissecting, Priscilla and Dan carried on a play of 'mother' and 'doctor',
> with the dead mice as children. They pretended to telephone to each
> other about it, saying, 'Your child is better now', and so on. Priscilla
> telephoned to Dan, 'Your child is cut in two'. Dan replied, 'Well,
> the best thing to do would be to put the two halves together again'.
> . . . Presently Dan said, 'Now I'm going to put some water on it, and
> make it come alive again'. Priscilla joined in this. . . . Priscilla gave
> Mrs. I. a dead mouse to hold, and said, 'Now it is alive again', and
> pretended to make it walk. Mrs. I. said, 'Is it?' Dan: 'Well, we are only
> pretending'.[22]

Eventually Isaacs persuaded Pyke to appoint a secretary to keep these
and other notes. In September 1926 Pyke also hired Nathan, who
had initially commuted to work in the City from Cambridge, to write
about the theory of knowledge. (Nathan's resulting essay was later
included as an appendix to Susan's first book about the school.[23])
In 1926 Pyke also hired as a teacher Dr Evelyn Lawrence, who
was to graduate later from the London School of Economics (LSE)
and became the second Mrs Isaacs, and in 1927 he also hired a
Russian-born teacher from New York, Richard Slavson, to teach
the children science. He had a film made about the school and on
24 July 1927 had it shown to a large audience in the Marble Arch
Pavilion, this resulting in widespread press coverage, including a
leader in *Nature*.[24]

But at the end of October 1927 Pyke's metal market investments
crashed. Meanwhile Susan had become increasingly irritated with

him for not leaving the running of the school to her, as he had originally agreed. By the end of 1927 she and Nathan had left. The school continued but it was plagued with financial difficulties, not helped by the failure of an appeal for funds to the Laura Spelman Rockefeller Trust signed by Sir Charles Sherrington, Cyril Burt, Jean Piaget, John Haldane, G. E. Moore and others. At the end of July 1929 the school closed. Twenty years later, after serving as a major figure in Mountbatten's team during the Second World War, Geoff Pyke committed suicide.

Malting House books

Pyke's Malting House project, however, lived on in Susan's numerous writings about its findings, including *Intellectual Growth in Young Children* (1930), which she dedicated to its pupils – her 'child companions'. She began by contrasting her approach with that of others – with the practical and scholarly approach, for instance, of Maria Montessori in her Maison des Petits in Geneva. She also took issue with the psychologist Piaget, who visited the school in 1927, and with whom she entered into critical academic debate over the next few years.[25]

Piaget held that children's development follows a step-wise sequence of stages. Isaacs, by contrast, argued that development involves a continuous process of increasing synthesis of children's knowledge and skills through their changing interests and phantasies. Adopting the example pioneered by Dewey in the USA, she described organizing her school to maximize the chance of young children pursuing whatever interested them and most immediately caught their imagination. Imagination and phantasy, she stressed, crucially bridge thought and reality. They inspire children to experiment and test the outer reality of their inner ideas. A case in point was her pupils' response to the death of the school's pet rabbit, which Isaacs noted thus in her diary:

> 14.7.25. . . . Dan found it and said, 'Its dead – its tummy does not move up and down now'. Paul said, 'My daddy says that if we put it into water, it will get alive again'. Mrs. I. said, 'Shall we do so and see?' They put it into a bath of water. Some of them said, 'It *is* alive'. It floated on the surface. One of them said, 'It's alive, because it's moving'. This was a circular movement, due to the current in the water. Mrs. I. therefore put in a small stick, which also moved round and round, and they agreed that the stick was not alive. They then suggested burying the rabbit, and all helped to dig a hole and bury it.[26]

Phantasy, Isaacs added, is also a starting-point for logic, as in the following example: 'Jessica (4;0) and Lena (4;2) were building castles in the sand, and told Mrs. I. that they were going to "build castles as high as the sky". But Jessica soon added, "If we did, the aeroplanes would knock them down" '.[27]

Bertrand Russell, in his book *The Scientific Outlook*, characterized Isaacs's approach as the 'application of psycho-analytic theory to education'.[28] But Isaacs disagreed. Her research, she said, was not educational but psychological. Above all, she emphasized, it was addressed to 'the desperate need of children themselves to be *understood*'[29] – a need she addressed further in her second Malting House book, *Social Development in Young Children*, published in 1933.

In it she again insisted that children's phantasies impel their scientific learning about the physical world around them.[30] She also insisted that phantasies impel children's learning about their social world. As support she cited the work of her fellow psychoanalyst Nina Searl. But most of all she cited the work of Melanie Klein, whom Pyke thought of approaching to analyse his son, and who had been to the school in 1925, during her lecture visit to London.

In her London lectures, included in *The Psycho-Analysis of Children* (1932), Klein gave examples of her child patients' phantasies of loving and hating, eating and biting. In her second Malting House book Isaacs gave more everyday, non-clinical examples. They included the following:

> 25.2.25. Harold had accidentally kicked Mrs. I.'s foot under the table, and this led him to say, 'I'll undress you and take off your suspenders, and gobble you all up' . . .
>
> 11.10.25. In the garden, Tommy ran after Mrs. I. and caught her. He said, 'I'll kill you,' and called Christopher and Penelope to 'come and help me push her down and kill her — and make her into ice-cream!' . . .
>
> 2.2.26. At lunch there was some talk about 'cutting Mrs. I. up' and 'having her for dinner'.[31]

Klein also described her patients' anal phantasies about faeces and urine. Again Isaacs provided more everyday examples, including:

> 19.11.24. At lunch the children had a conversation as to what people were 'made of', and spoke of people being made of pudding, pie, potatoes, coal, etc., and of 'bee-wee', 'try', 'do-do', 'ah-ah', 'bottie'. . . .
>
> 24.11.24. Frank said, 'and poison him'. And another time, 'and make spots come out all over him'.[32]

Reporting her analysis of her four-year-old son, Erich, and of her six-year-old patient, Erna, Klein gave examples of children's phantasies about their parents and grownups generally (see pp. 15–16 above). Again Isaacs provided examples of similar phantasies:

16.1.25. While modelling, Frank said, apropos of a long piece of plasticine, 'Somebody's climbing up the lady's ah-ah [lavatory] house' . . .

2.2.26. The children said they were 'going to have a wedding', and there was much talk as to whether Priscilla would marry Frank or Dan. . . . Frank said, 'You *can't* marry Dan, because daddy must be bigger than mammy'. . . . [W]e asked each child in turn whether his mammy or his daddy was the bigger. Christopher reported quite accurately that his mammy was; but Dan denied this of C.'s parents . . . [and] said, stamping his foot, 'Yes, you see, I *shall* be bigger than Priscilla', thus twisting Frank's argument to suit his own phantasy.

13.12.26. While Jane, Conrad and Dan were drawing with crayons, Conrad asked Jane whether she had 'seen Dan's mummie's penis' – but at once corrected himself and said, 'No, she hasn't got one. Have you seen her overs?' (ovaries? vulva?). Jane replied, 'No, I haven't, but I've seen my mummie's'. Conrad: 'So've I'.[33]

Isaacs was warned against publishing these and other observations lest they damage her reputation. Other observations were less contentious: her pupils' phantasies, for instance, about making what Isaacs called 'cosy places', phantasies which she claimed signified children's longing to protect their inner world from outside danger and attack, as in the following example: '5.2.26. The elder children arranged chairs and tables round themselves in the summer-house, while they were modelling, "to keep the tigers out". They asked Mrs. I. to "be a tiger and come" – and to "come from a distance, so that we can hear you growling"'.[34]

Klein attributed her child patients' phantasies about similar 'growling' figures in their external world to fears about their parents as punishing superego figures within them. Again Isaacs provided more everyday examples, such as:

8.10.24. The children were standing at the door, watching a heavy shower of rain. They heard the rustling noise of the rain on the leaves, and when something was said about this, George remarked, 'Perhaps it's God saying He will punish us for doing things we shouldn't'. . . .

20.1.25. After the children had played Harold's game of running round the room, saying that they were 'going to blow up' the tower of bricks which he had built, they presently asked Mrs. I. to say, 'I'm going to tell the policeman'; and soon Frank begged her to 'go and *pretend* to tell the policeman'.[35]

Klein provided numerous instances of similar anxiety-inducing phantasies of destroying things. She less often described children's more constructive and happier phantasies – perhaps because, as Isaacs observed, 'The happiest days with children, as the happiest women's lives, are those that have no history'.[36] She sought to make good this oversight. She recounted examples of her pupils' phantasies of love and generous concern for others, as in the following incidents:

> 25.11.24. Dan's father came into the school room, and sat down beside Dan and Benjie, who were modelling. Benjie asked him, 'What have you come for, Mr. X.?' 'To talk to you and Mrs. I.' Benjie made a basket with eggs in it, and gave it to Mr. X. Then he made a motor boat and gave that to him, and then another basket. . . .

> 10.12.24. Harold and Benjie were pushing the large table to the other side of the room, and accidentally bumped Paul with it. Paul flung himself on the floor crying. . . . Harold ran to get his own handkerchief for Paul, and sat down beside Paul with his hand on Paul's head, comforting him. He kissed him, and sat by him until Paul stopped crying and got up. . . .

> 23.3.25. Dan cried at lunch-time because he had not been given a brown plate, and when Harold, who had a brown plate, had finished his pudding, he took his spoon off and passed it to Dan – 'You can have my brown plate.' He stroked his hand affectionately several times, and Dan said to him, 'I love you, Harold, I love you.' . . .

> 4.6.26. When Priscilla shut Dan up as a 'puppy', and he began to cry with boredom, Alfred said to him, 'Don't cry, Dan – I'll be your nurse,' and Priscilla agreed.[37]

Other examples came from Isaacs's work after leaving Cambridge in 1927 for London, where she and Nathan then settled in 16c Primrose Hill Road, NW3 – a flat in which Marion Milner later recalled Susan's interest in phantasy involving inviting guests to play charades, and from which Susan increasingly became involved in teaching, writing and advising about children and their phantasies.

Teaching, writing and advising

In 1927, on her return to London, Susan went into analysis with Joan Riviere, partly to learn more about Klein's work. She remained in analysis with Riviere until 1933 and dedicated *Social Development in Young Children* to her. The book added to her reputation as a child development adviser, as did her work lecturing at Morley College and at UCL, where Cyril Burt also employed her to supervise his advanced psychology students. She also gave public lectures, including one on 27 June 1927 for the British Psychological Society, in which she defended Klein's method of child analysis against that of Anna Freud. Just as Klein emphasized the early disjunction between children's inner image of their parents and their parents' outer behaviour, and the way this disjunction contributes to neurosis, so too did Isaacs.[38] Isaacs added that children often construe the losses involved in weaning and potty-training in phantasy terms: outer figures constructed out of inner figures punish them for imagining destroying their mothers by biting and eating them, or by robbing them of their faeces.[39]

Isaacs also gave radio talks and wrote popular books about children's phantasies. The latter included *The Nursery Years* (1929), which *The Times* praised as 'a classic of popular exposition'.[40] It contains an engaging description of the inner meaning the baby gives to his outer experience:

> He not only eats, but thinks with his mouth . . . [W]e can see too that the baby *loves* with his mouth, and feels his mother's love in her gift of the breast. . . . But if the mother withdraws the breast how quicky the picture changes! His face puckers and reddens, he screams with distress and anger, his fists clench and his body stiffens in protest. . . . Thus are little children in these critical early years torn and tossed between their loves and their hates, between the delights of possession and the fears and anxieties of loss.[41]

The Nursery Years was followed by a book about primary school-children called *The Children We Teach*.[42] Isaacs dedicated it to Klein and Searl, and included examples gleaned both from her Malting House work and from articles about seven- to eleven-year-olds which she had contributed to the magazine *Teacher's World*. Both books became a major influence on education policy in England and abroad through the ensuing decade.[43]

Between 1929 and 1936 Isaacs also popularized Klein's ideas in answering readers' letters to the magazine *Nursery World*, in which she covered children's phantasies about where babies come from, smacking, masturbation, reading, writing and so on. Nathan suggested she adopt the pen name Ursula Wise, which she duly did. Ursula was also the name she gave to the only child she described at length in her second Malting House book, focusing on the phantasies Ursula used in dealing inwardly with the outward fact of her mother bearing and giving birth to her younger sister when Ursula was four, just as Susan had had to deal with the birth of her younger sister, Alice, when she too was four.[44]

Besides her writing activities, Susan was chair from 1928 to 1931 of the Education Section of the British Psychological Society, and served on the editorial boards of the *British Journal of Educational*

Psychology (from 1931) and of the *British Journal of Medical Psychology* (from 1936). In 1931 she was appointed a psychologist on the staff of the London Clinic of Psycho-Analysis. Concurrently she again worked for the WEA, this time running a class at Toynbee Hall, which she gave to Marion Milner (who needed the money because her husband was too ill to work) when she became head of England's first university-based child development department in 1993. It complemented those already run by Piaget in Geneva, by Arnold Gesell in New Haven, and by Bott in Toronto.

Designing the post for her, the director of London University's Institute of Education, Sir Percy Nunn, insisted it was essential to appoint an 'able and qualified woman' who could both teach and inspire research.[45] Susan was initially uncertain whether to take the post but finally accepted it on 11 May 1933. Her new department began that autumn with five full-time students. Lecturers included Donald Winnicott, who also provided a student placement in his outpatient department at Paddington Green Children's Hospital. Isaacs added other clinic and nursery school placements as well as educational visits, including a visit in the spring of 1934 to Dartington Hall's progressive school.[46]

During the 1930s Susan also provided child development advice to government departments. In answering an enquiry about fairy tales from an inspector at the Board of Education, she dwelt on their mixed benefits: they externalize children's 'phantasies in a form that robs them of their individual terror', but they also risk seeming to make real what the child dreads.[47] She also gave lectures on similar issues at the Institute of Psycho-Analysis: in 1934, for example, she talked about ways children become defiant, as she had been as a child, to protect themselves against wanting anything from their mothers.[48] Other reasons for children to become defiant, she said, are: that they feel they have insufficient goodness inside to put right, or to take responsibility for putting right, actual or imagined damage they have done to their mothers; that they imagine their mothers as hateful and bad and as therefore fully warranting their attacking them; that they use defiance to test whether their parents are as bad as they imagine them to be; that they defy their parents to confess and bring to their parents' attention the bad people they feel themselves to be; or that they are defiant to make themselves look as big and powerful outwardly as they inwardly imagine their parents to be.

In 1934 Isaacs also spoke to a symposium of the Medical Section of the British Psychological Society (of which she was the first non-medical woman committee member) about children's phantasies of greedily robbing and enviously spoiling what is inside their mothers.[49] In another talk she dwelt on what she called children's 'bad habits'

– thumb-sucking, masturbation and so on – habits she analysed in terms of children's phantasies of having their sexually coupling parents inside them.[50]

As well as analysing children's ills she was also now beginning to suffer all too real ills herself. In December 1935 she was treated for cancer with radium. It in turn led to her suffering pleurisy-like symptoms the next month. Undaunted, however, she continued to be immensely hard-working, including compiling a teachers' record card system in 1936 for Wiltshire's education committee.[51] Helped by Ilse Hellman,[52] a recently arrived developmental psychology graduate from Vienna, she continued to answer readers' letters to *Nursery World*. She also answered readers' letters to *Home and School*, a magazine edited by George Lyward, who later went on to run a progressive school for delinquent teenagers, and for whom she also edited a number of pamphlets.[53] And in 1937 she gave lectures in New Zealand and Australia and was awarded an honorary DSc in Adelaide. During the late 1930s she also edited a series of books entitled Contributions to Modern Education.[54] And in the autumn of 1938, after being rehoused with the Institute of Education in London University's new Senate House building, Isaacs's child development department reopened with much of its playroom furniture supplied by Paul Abbatt, to whose father she had run away from home when she was six. Despite her illness, she continued work as a child analyst.

Child analysis

Child analysis provided Isaacs with yet more examples of children's phantasies. They included those of a three-and-a-half-year-old boy, whom I will call Colin, whom Isaacs described in a talk to the Education Section of the British Psychological Society in 1934.[55] Referred for treatment because he was so dirty and given to violent temper tantrums, Colin felt that his tantrums were to blame for a succession of fourteen nurses leaving him: his first nurse left when he was one and his younger brother was born. To control his outward behaviour he got Isaacs to bind a wooden doll tightly round and round with string and paper, symbolically to stop him screaming and dirtying himself and driving her and his current nurse away over the Christmas break.

Another example involved a four-year-old, Jack, also referred because of temper tantrums. His tantrums, it turned out, had various causes: he could be screaming for his father (who had died from TB when he was a baby) to come and help his mother in her hard life bringing him up alone; he could be identifying with his father as an alive, loud and violent figure; or he could be making an inward attack on his father for being 'bad' in not being alive and available to help his mother. Perhaps Isaacs was also thinking of Jack in her talk at the Paris congress of 1938,[56] when she described a boy's phantasy about his mother attacking him being lessened through verbalizing his phantasy. Certainly she talked about Jack in another talk in 1938 – to the British Psycho-Analytical Society – in which she described him putting one toy train coach in front and another behind an engine, and then anxiously and repeatedly asking, 'Engines *do* go like this, don't they?'[57] She linked this with his living with 'one Daddy and two Mummies' (his uncle, aunt and mother) and with his image of his mother as dominant and anti-men with her insistence that ladies go first. When Isaacs thus verbalized his fear of his mother she apparently became a less harsh, more benign figure in his mind.

In a second paper to the Paris congress of 1938,[58] Isaacs returned to the example of Colin to further illustrate children's inward re-presentation of figures in their outer world. She described Colin's tantrums as means by which he attacked an inner image of his mother. In one of his treatment sessions, he ate some sugar and then took a ball of plasticine and got her to make the plasticine into lots of little balls corresponding to the number of patterned daisies on her dress. It represented his phantasy, she said, of eating her up as he had eaten the sugar, whereupon, fearing she might retaliate by eating him up, he sought to allay his fear by externalizing it through getting her to punish and drag him around the room at the end of a skipping-rope.

Isaacs spoke more about Colin at a talk to the London Institute of Psycho-Analysis (7 December 1938) attended by Anna Freud and her colleagues Dorothy Burlingham and Marie Bonaparte. Criticized for being too condensed,[59] Isaacs expanded her talk for its publication in 1940 to include further examples, for instance the phantasy she had first described in 1923, in which a four-and-a-half-year-old girl had been impelled to swallow her envied older brother's whistle. She also noted that children seek to control those they envy, love and fear by imagining they are 'taking them in'.

Isaacs went on to reiterate this theme in a talk in Paris (30 April 1939) to British and French psychoanalysts. She took up Melanie Klein's 'depressive position' theory that we control figures in our minds so as to defend ourselves against dependence on them and against loss of their outward counterparts. Analysis, she claimed, lib-erates children from these inwardly controlled and controlling figures through attending to their good and constructive feelings as well as bad and destructive ones. 'What we are always concerned with in our work', she added, is the inner '*meaning to the child* of the person in question or the external events which impinge upon him' (emphasis in original).[60]

In another paper she emphasized a related theme: how children and adults control their inner world by enacting it outwardly.[61] She illustrated the point with the case of a fifteen-year-old who, following his parents' separation when he was seven, lived with his grandmother whom his mother now bitterly criticized in trying to persuade him to come and live with her. In his analysis he externalized the phantasy to which this gave rise. He became preoccupied with making a parachute attached to a basket in which he planned to gently lower the family cat from an upstairs window. He thereby represented externally an image he could not bear internally of vomiting out his grandmother made bad by his mother's criticisms of her. Or so Isaacs said. She added that by verbalizing children's phantasies the analyst helps to restore an otherwise severed link between the child's inner and outer reality.

Evacuation and war

Outer reality again included war. It took Susan's husband, Nathan, to Warwickshire, where his involvement in ensuring Britain's wartime supply of tungsten and molybdenum earned him an OBE. Meanwhile – just a short cycle ride and two changes of train away – Susan lived briefly in Cambridge, where she shared a home with Sibyl Clement Brown, a colleague at the LSE, which was now evacuated there from London. Susan found them a flat and became involved from autumn 1939 until spring 1940 with Clement Brown, R. H. Thouless, John Bowlby and others in investigating the effects on children of being evacuated from Tottenham and Islington in North London to Cambridge, as happened to three thousand children in the early months of the war.

In her report Isaacs criticized the authorities for being so concerned with such outer details as train timetables and housing, overlooking the inner psychological effects on the children involved.[62] To highlight these effects she quoted the children in their own words, including an eight-year-old who wrote: 'I miss my tortoise in LanDon he is Robert Taylor he bit me once he bit me. And I tod [told] him he wac [was] a note [naughty] boy and I fod [fed] him a lost [lots] of tam [times]'. She also quoted a fifteen-year-old girl who wrote: 'I miss my relations, parents and friends who are in Tottenham. And I often wish our foster mother wasn't so particular'.[63]

Meanwhile Susan was briefly joined in her own evacuation to Cambridge by Klein, before the latter's move to Pitlochry and

Susan's return in 1941 to London, where the Ministry of Education urged her to reopen her child development department. She negotiated for her post there to be made full-time but then found someone else – one of her department's first students, Dorothy Gardner – to fill it. She continued to give lectures in the department. But the wartime work for which she is best known in psychoanalysis was her defence of Klein against her detractors in the British Psycho-Analytical Society's Controversial Discussions.

Her defence began on 27 January 1943 with a discussion of her pre-circulated essay, 'The nature and function of phantasy'. It constituted the culmination of the work she had done in previous years in drawing attention to children's phantasies. She reiterated Klein's extension of Freud's concept of phantasy beyond dreams to include everything mediating between inner and outer reality. But she also went further: she insisted on the ubiquity of phantasy. 'There is no impulse, no instinctual urge', she declared, 'which is not experienced as (unconscious) phantasy'.[64] Phantasy, she insisted, involves the sexual impulses described by Freud. It also involves the destructive impulses, anxieties and inner–outer defences of introjection and projection described by Klein. She rejected the claim of Robert Wälder, Anna Freud and other psychoanalysts from Vienna that inner phantasy representation of our parents is limited to superego figures beginning with the Oedipal conflicts of late infancy. Rather, she maintained, phantasy extends into earliest infancy. After all, she pointed out, Freud himself noted that, by the age of eighteen months, his grandson already had an inner phantasy of his mother which he represented externally as a spool of thread he variously threw away and retrieved as means of dealing with her going away and his wanting her to come back.

To this example Isaacs added others she had learnt about from her work as a headmistress, analyst, journalist, child development researcher and policy adviser, for example:

> A litte girl of one year 6 months saw a shoe of her mother's from which the sole had come loose and was flapping about. The child was horrified and screamed with terror. . . . At two years and 11 months (15 months later), she suddenly said in a frightened voice to her mother 'Where are Mummy's broken shoes?' Her mother hastily said, fearing another screaming attack, that she had sent them away. The child then commented, 'They might have eaten me right up!'[65]

The little girl's comment, Isaacs maintained, indicated that at eighteen months she already had a phantasy, which she could not yet express in words, that her mother's shoes might eat her up. This phantasy, Isaacs claimed, stemmed from a still earlier phantasy of her mother retaliating against her wanting to bite and eat her up by biting her.

In 1929 Isaacs had described a similar phantasy in *The Nursery Years*, of a fourteen-month-old toddler waking up terrified of a white rabbit biting him.[66] Now, in the essay, she linked the same child's biting phantasy to a game he had played a couple of months later, in which he shouted 'Quack, quack' as he shooed imaginary ducks into the corner of the room. By shooing them and their enormous beaks away, Isaacs wrote, he sought to quell his earlier white rabbit nightmare. This in turn was the product of a still earlier phantasy of his mother biting him in revenge for his wanting to bite her – a phantasy evident, said Isaacs, in his rejecting and refusing the milk his mother gave him on weaning him at seven months.

As further evidence of the ubiquity and early appearance of children's phantasies, Isaacs returned to an example she had used in a talk promoting nursery school education.[67] In another contribution to the British Psycho-Analytical Society's Controversial Discussions, which she wrote with Paula Heimann (who later recalled Susan working so closely with her husband, Nathan, they even shared the same double desk),[68] the example is detailed further:

> A girl of sixteen months often plays her favourite game with her parents. She picks small imaginary bits off a brown embossed leather screen in the dining-room, carrying these pretended bits of food across the room in her finger and thumb and putting them into the mouth of father and mother alternately. She chooses the brown screen, with small raised lumps on it . . . to represent the 'food' she wishes to give her parents.[69]

The little girl thereby turned into a pleasurable game, according to Heimann and Isaacs, the anxiety and guilt she felt, aged twelve to sixteen months, at being told off by her parents for smearing herself with her faeces and putting them into her mouth while lying in her cot in the morning.

Argument continued in the British Psycho-Analytical Society as to whether such examples constitute evidence of the early occurrence of phantasy. Meanwhile Isaacs served from 1946 on the Training Committee of the London Institute of Psycho-Analysis, as a member of the its Board from 1945 to 1947 and on the Council of the London Clinic of Psycho-Analysis from 1946. She also continued writing in support of Klein,[70] as well as contributing articles and government memoranda on a number of child development and policy issues. One of these pleaded for a better understanding of children's response to losing their fathers – through their death or absence – during the war.[71] She argued strongly against children being brought up away from home in a memo described by one authority as the 'most important single document' consulted by the government's Curtiss Committee in deciding postwar childcare policy.[72] Her memo ended with yet another phantasy, that of a fifteen-year-old orphaned servant who, Isaacs wrote, filled a drawer with photos she stole from her employers in order to satisfy her inner 'longing to be a member of a family and to have kind and loving parents and brothers and sisters of her own'.[73]

Isaacs's memo including this example was published in 1945. That winter the Isaacses' Primrose Hill flat was bombed. Shortly afterwards, still ill with the cancer that had first afflicted her in 1935, Susan suffered pneumonia.[74] In January 1946 she gave up the teaching she had undertaken at the LSE, and stopped teaching at the Institute of Education. In her last public lecture she paid tribute to Grace Owen, who had introduced her at Manchester University to the progressive education ideas of Dewey; Isaacs had done much to develop these ideas in highlighting the importance of phantasy in children's lives. In late 1947 she underwent surgery for removal of an ulcer. She was made a CBE in the New Year's honours list of 1948.[75]

Troubles of Children, Isaacs's last childcare advice book, was published in 1948, as were her collected papers, *Childhood and After*, and a revised version of her seminal essay about phantasy for the *International Journal of Psycho-Analysis*. In the revision she was helped by Nathan's niece, Karina, who had stayed with them in Cambridge and Warwickshire during the war. The essay included yet more examples of children's phantasies, including one recounted by Ernest Jones of a small boy who, seeing his mother breastfeed the new baby, exclaimed 'That's what you bit me with'.[76]

With this her major contribution in noting and publicizing the ubiquity of children's phantasies ended. After holidaying that summer in the Scottish Highlands, where her mother had grown up, she died at home on 12 October 1948. On the day of her death she told her one-time student and colleague Dorothy Gardner of her life-long quest for understanding. It was the counterpart of children's longing to be understood of which she had so often written. It was this longing that had driven her to investigate and draw attention to ways we all use phantasy to bridge inner and outer reality. Her analyst and colleague Joan Riviere, the subject of my next chapter, had by this time begun to explore the inner world concealed by outward masquerades of what is now known as gender.

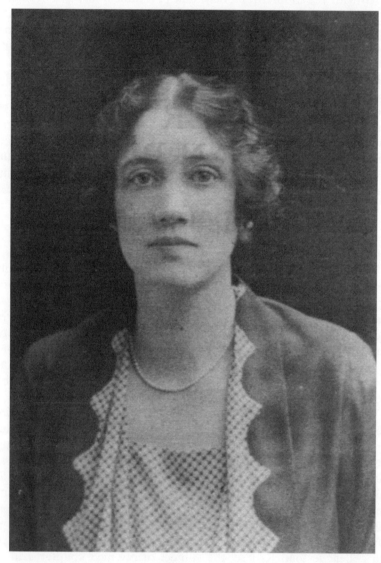

Joan Riviere, *c*.1928

3 Joan Riviere: Gendered Masquerades

Although Susan Isaacs's major importance lies in her discoveries about children's phantasies, her account of them is sometimes rather unimaginative, flat, even cold. Joan Riviere's is, by contrast, eloquent and evocative. Its stylishness is consistent with her attention to outward appearance and her Bloomsbury society background. This in turn arguably contributed to the insights for which she is best known: those regarding womanliness, and gender generally, as not necessarily given by an inner essence, but as also functioning as an outer mask or 'masquerade'. Beyond such masquerading she also importantly depicted the destructive envy, emptiness and depressive gloom which can occur in men and women. First, though, what of these factors in her own early womanhood?

Early femininity[1]

Riviere's early years were spent in Sussex, where her family had for many generations enjoyed high social standing and literary connections. One of her forebears wrote a cookery book owned and annotated by Thomas Grey. Another was a bookseller. Several served as 'masters' of the White Hart inn near Glyndebourne.[2] Her uncle Arthur Verral was a distinguished Classics don at Cambridge. His lectures were the only ones worth attending, her psychoanalyst colleague James Strachey later recalled. Strachey also noted Verral's distinction in being the first to demonstrate that Euripides' play *Alcestis* was written to counter the religious hypocrisy and cant of his day, just as Riviere, in her writing, exposed the frequent hypocrisy of outward show and masquerading.

Joan's father, Hugh John Verral, was a solicitor, and less distinguished than Arthur, while her mother, Anna Hodgson, came from a much less grand family. Born in 1854, Anna was the third of fourteen children of a Devonshire parson. She took the Cambridge Higher Women's Examinations in 1877, and worked for six years as a governess in England and Gibraltar before marrying and settling with Hugh Verral in Brighton.

Their first child was born on 9 July 1882, but he survived only a few hours. Joan was born on 28 June 1883. Then came another girl – Mary, known as Molly – born on 18 April 1885, followed two years later by the birth of Cuthbert. When Joan was four her mother started teaching her to read, and when she was six she started formal education. This included drawing lessons at the local art school from when she was eight, and violin lessons from when she was nine. Meanwhile her mother despaired of Cuthbert. She wrote of him as a 'poor boy' with 'curvature of the spine and his feet are not right', and, at five, as 'still rather a baby and learning nothing from lessons'.[3]

Joan's own learning took her to boarding school, Wycombe Abbey, in Buckinghamshire, where she stayed until she was seventeen. Her mother despaired of her too. She described her as 'not well' on leaving school. Nevertheless she arranged for her soon to leave home again – this time to stay with a Fräulein Metzeroth in Gotha where, for the next year, Joan learnt German and continued to study the violin and painting. On her return to England she lived in a bed and breakfast at 43 Belsize Park in north-west London, worked as a court dressmaker with a firm called Nettleship, travelled in England and abroad, and attended various high society events, including weddings, debutante balls and private views of art exhibitions. Anna was proud of her social success. But she also criticized her as 'still very lacking in softness and lovable qualities at home'. And she mentioned that others, for example her grandmother, would describe her as 'impressive', but as also having an 'unconscious air of superiority'.[4]

Whatever her outward appearance, Joan was inwardly unwell. She wrote of her interest in psychology, in connection with a novel by Paul Heyse, to a Herr Bode in Germany. And she consulted a number of doctors on account of various ills. She also had in-patient treatment in March and September 1902 when, with the advice of a Dr Griffin, she underwent minor surgery, possibly gynaecological. Meanwhile she continued her involvement in London's smart Bloomsbury set in which she figured, according to James Strachey, as 'tall, strikingly handsome, distinguished-looking, and somehow impressive'.[5] In her early twenties she married a Chancery barrister, Evelyn Riviere, the son of a then famous Royal Academician painter, Briton Riviere. Their marriage took place on 14 July 1906 at St Peter's in Brighton, after which they set up home in a flat in a Georgian house, 16 York Place, in a fashionable area of London near Regent's Park. Here Joan's sister, Molly, often stayed, and the Rivieres entertained, and went to concerts and parties. They went for holidays both abroad and in England, where they stayed variously in Cambridge, Mundesley, with Joan's parents in Brighton, and with Evelyn's parents in Flaxley.

In 1907 Joan started getting involved in women's suffrage meetings. The next February her brother Cuthbert emigrated to Canada. And on 7 June 1908 Joan gave birth to her only child, Diana. The next spring Joan was suddenly called to Brighton, where her father, long ill with rheumatic fever, died on 19 March 1909. Within the week she was back in London, going to the theatre, meetings and dinner parties and continuing her dressmaking work. In April 1910 she moved with Evelyn and Diana to 10 Nottingham Terrace. John Addington Symonds's granddaughter, Katharine West, later remembered her from this time in nearby Regent's Park, close to the Wests' Sussex Place home, as a 'tall, Edwardian beauty with a picture hat and scarlet parasol – walking up and down the seashell path in lively conversation with a gentleman'.[6] Social and leisure-time engagements included meeting Anna Pavlova in May 1910, going to art exhibitions, the opera and ballet (including seeing Nijinsky in March 1913), reading recently published controversial novels (D. H. Lawrence's *The Rainbow*, for instance), going to psychology lectures and learning Russian. She also attended meetings of Roger Fry's Omega Workshops which, like the nineteenth-century Arts and Crafts movement inspired by William Morris, sought to apply developments in art to the design of ordinary household goods such as furniture, pottery and textiles.

From 1913 she also became involved in the Medico-Psychological Society. Led by the novelist May Sinclair and others, that year the society founded the first clinic to make psychoanalytic treatment available to the general public. Joan was by now in treatment. Following her father's death she had suffered a number of minor ailments – insomnia, gastritis, colds, flu and styes. In 1910 she broke down completely and sought psychiatric help, including eleven consultations, in early 1915, with a 'mental specialist' called Wright (whom Leonard Woolf also consulted when he was worried about his wife, Virginia).

It is unlikely that Joan met Virginia Woolf, but she certainly met her sister and brother-in-law, Vanessa and Clive Bell. She also met

Lady Ottoline Morrell, the artists Walter Sickert and Walter Lamb and the writers Enid Bagnold and E. M. Forster. And she sat for the artists Gerald Kelly and R. G. Eaves who, in 1916, drew a picture of her that is still in the family. In January 1916 her brother Cuthbert, then serving in a Canadian regiment, returned briefly to England. On 19 February 1916, having long been interested in psychoanalysis, she consulted Ernest Jones and a couple of days later went into analysis with him.

Jones and Freud

Joan saw Jones at 12.30 p.m. each day. Evidently they got on well. Not long after her analysis began, he lent her his country cottage, The Plat, in Elstead, Surrey, from 29 July to 8 August 1916, and again from 18 December 1916 to 22 January 1917. The next month he married a Welsh musician who was very much younger than him. Some months earlier Joan had decided to go into a sanatorium, stayed in Norbach nursing home that April, and in July 1917 went to a London nursing home for an operation on her nose. Having thus interrupted her analysis for several months, she resumed it in late September 1917 and continued until mid-April 1918, when Jones broke it off. A few months later, on 8 September 1918, she received a telegram saying that his wife was dead – from a suddenly abcessed appendix for which Jones had summoned help to no avail from the London surgeon Wilfred Trotter. Joan wrote to Jones the next month:

> I regard it as absolutely unquestionable that your wife was to you a substitute for me . . . it had been quite clear that you *expected* to be happy in your marriage, and I with great difficulty constrained myself to resuming the analysis (because it was my only means to a knowledge of psycho-analysis which I felt was bound up with my interest in life) under the expectation that your feeling for me in the future would be simply one of friendly indifference. What was my astonishment when I got back after 6 months to find, not this, but a formality and impersonality in you that amounted to 'hardness' quite brutal in *my* then 'quivering' and 'wounded' state.[7]

A few days later she complained that he had driven her to the verge of suicide, just as she had similarly been driven by two men eight years before. Jones agreed at the end of 1918 to see her again as a patient. Soon he also referred patients to her. And, following his reorganization and founding of the British Psycho-Analytical Society in 1919, she became a founder member on 10 April 1919.

The first issue of the *International Journal of Psycho-Analysis* (1920) included one of Riviere's translations of Freud, his essay of 1917,

'One of the difficulties of psychoanalysis'. Later in 1920 the journal also carried a brief clinical note by her.[8] Written in her mid-thirties, it focused on the three-cornered relationships of a twenty-eight-year-old patient who dreamt she heard burglars and that two people were asleep together. The dream reminded her patient of how, when she was six, a young man had assaulted her, and of how she had wanted to take her mother's and then her stepmother's place in marrying her father. Perhaps it was a similar wish in Joan to take the place of Jones's wife that led him again to break off her analysis in June 1921; his second marriage, to Katherine Jokl, had taken place on 9 October 1919.

Although Jones stopped seeing Joan as a patient, they continued meeting through their joint involvement in the Glossary Committee, which included the Stracheys and met in Jones's house to work on translating Freud. Joan's translation work now involved editing Freud's *Collected Papers* and retranslating (with Jones and Flügel) Freud's *Introductory Lectures on Psycho-Analysis* of 1916–17. Freud was evidently impressed. He wrote to her in the summer of 1919 saying that if, as seemed possible, she wanted analysis with him she would 'take precedence over everyone else, as my translator and as an outstanding member of the London group'.[9]

Jones warned him that she was 'a case of typical hysteria, almost the only symptoms being sexual anaesthesia and unorganized Angst, with a few inhibitions'. He also confessed to Freud his error in lending Joan his country cottage. It had provoked her to declare her love and to react to his rejection with the 'broken-hearted cry that she had never been rejected before', he wrote, adding that she had been the mistress of several men, and that since his rejection of her, 'she devoted herself to torturing me without any intermission and with considerable success and ingenuity, being a fiendish sadist'. He had, he said, been unable to master her negative transference. But she was much improved, could now talk fluently at meetings, whereas before she had been 'dumb with Angst'. He ended, however, by describing her as having the 'most colossal narcissism imaginable . . . a strong complex about being a well-born lady (county family)' that went with her despising 'all the rest of us, especially the women'.[10]

Freud was less hostile. He began treating her in Vienna on 25 February 1922 and a month later wrote to Jones: 'Mrs. Riviere does not appear to me half as black as you had painted her. We agree nicely so far. Maybe the difficulties will come later. In my experience you have not to scratch too deeply the skin of a so called masculine woman to bring her femininity to the light'.[11] But Jones went on complaining, in particular that she wanted to become the *Inter-*

national Journal's 'translating editor'. Freud supported her request, while acknowledging that she could be difficult – 'a concentrated acid', he wrote, 'not to be used until duly diluted'.[12] But Jones went on bridling at her superior attitude. Freud explained it as a mask for inner unhappiness. With him too, he wrote, she was 'harsh, unpleasant, critical even'. But it turned out, he went on, that this was a cover for inner unease:

> She cannot tolerate praise, triumph and success, not any better than failure, blame and repudiation. . . . To be sure this conflict, which is the cause of her continuous dissatisfaction, is not known to her consciousness; whenever it is revived she projects her self-criticism to other people, turns her pangs of conscience into sadistic behaviour, tries to render other people unhappy because she feels so herself. . . . Her sexual freedom may be an appearance, the keeping up of which required those conspicuous compensatory attitudes as haughtiness, majestic behaviour etc.[13]

In his book *The Ego and the Id* (1923), which Riviere later translated, and which was based on a talk he gave to the Berlin congress of September 1922, Freud wrote generally about such patients. He described them reacting with unease, discontent and invariable worsening of their condition when the analyst talks hopefully about their getting better.[14] But this did not stop him being hopeful about Joan. During the holiday break in her treatment in August 1922 he wrote to Jones: 'The good impression she has made on me did not vanish with her personal presence'.[15] And he wrote the next month to Joan hoping she would now 'be better able to bear a word of appreciation in private'.[16]

But she remained intolerant of praise, and turned her intolerance against others, particularly against women, as Jones had noted. On arriving in Vienna in October 1922 for six weeks' further analysis with Freud, for instance, she wrote to her sister and mother decrying the women she had met on the way: 'I got my sleeper all right in the train, but another woman was shoved in on top – I always seem to have the same type in sleepers, common little actresses in fur coats, very much made-up, and covered with scent. However they always are rather cringing and seem to realize my superior claims'. She similarly deplored a railway booking clerk in Berlin, referring to her as 'a very disagreeable German young woman, who never spoke or looked at one, like a post office attendant, so that you never know if she hears or understands what you want, or whether she is doing your business or going on with someone else's'.[17] Freud regretted her snobbery. Her analysis with him having ended in November 1922, he wrote to her the following January, saying he wished he could have gone on treating her so as to show her the link between her neurosis and her 'national or social prejudice'.[18]

Continuing snobbery

Riviere's snobbery persisted. So did her contempt. In 1921–2 she wrote the first of a number of book reviews and clinical notes, often eloquent but often high-handedly dismissive in tone. She decried one writer's book about psychoanalysis as 'one of the legion of popular works on this subject that are now falling from the press like leaves in autumn'.[19] She declared another 'trivial', typical of the 'hypocritical English' and 'characteristic of the stream of little manuals on psycho-analysis now being published'.[20] Yet another she scorned as 'pernicious nonsense' with its insistence that analysts should be violent and forceful in giving their interpretations 'with a steel fist'.[21]

One of the clinical notes ridiculed those who, believing their dreams to be 'extraordinary', bore others with them at breakfast. She took dreams seriously, however, and reported those of her patients about grand people and places. One dreamt her father had a moustache like the Kaiser's. Another dreamt he and the Prince of Wales were plying a lady with 'Imperial Beauties'. Still another dreamt of a beautiful cathedral: it reminded him of how, when he was seven, he went to a small country church, where he used to adore a 'beautiful little girl much superior to him in social position'[22] – perhaps an allusion to Joan. After this case, Riviere at last produced an appreciative review – of Strachey's translation of Freud's *Group Psychology and the Analysis of the Ego*. She commended it for overcoming 'our English shyness in matters of sex' so often resulting in what she called 'an almost insuperable difficulty in expressing ourselves at all, outside poetry, on anything relating to the emotions'.[23]

The review was published in 1923. In July that year Freud wrote to her of the death of his four-year-old grandson, Heinz, the previous month: 'You may perhaps remember him', Freud added, 'he came running into the room once during your treatment, I showed him to you and later he asked several times about the "tall auntie"'.[24] Perhaps it was partly in memory of the little boy's death that she sent Freud a book that Christmas about Tutankhamen's tomb. Freud replied shortly afterwards by having flowers sent to her: she had just had an operation for fibroids.

Riviere's abrasive reviews continued with a sarcastic account of a book about the psychology of fashion.[25] As for her clinical publications, they now included three vignettes: one about a woman who imagined her husband's penis as bruised, bloody and mangled, and Riviere kissing it so her lips also became covered with blood;[26] another about a patient regaling her with an anecdote about her three-year-old son threatening to break off his penis, and imagining her giving birth through her 'seat';[27] and a patient dismissing lesbianism as 'boring . . . pointless . . . meaningless – like trying to play tennis without balls!'[28] But it is for her next clinical publication, 'Womanliness as a masquerade' (1929), that she is now best known, at least within feminist theory.[29]

Gendered masquerades

In 'Womanliness as a masquerade' Riviere explicitly cited, for the first time, the work of Melanie Klein. They had met in 1920 at the Hague congress, had holidayed together in the Endelberg after the Bad Homburg congress of 1921 and had become still more friendly at the Salzburg congress of 1924. It is possible that in 1924 Riviere also attended the meeting at Würzburg, where Klein presented her paper about her six-year-old patient Erna. Certainly she attended Klein's lectures in London in July 1925. The same year Klein joined Joan and her family on holiday in Switzerland. When Klein decided to live in England in 1926, Riviere wrote her a letter of welcome, also offering a room in her aunt Verral's house.

Meanwhile her friendship with Freud was cooling. She was irritated at his asking someone else to translate his book *Inhibitions, Symptoms and Anxiety* (1926). Freud in turn was irritated with her because of her contribution to the London symposium in May 1927, at which she had supported Klein's version of child analysis against that of his daughter, Anna. Against Anna's insistence on differences between child and adult analysis, Joan insisted on their similarities. In both cases, she said, the patient's manifest wish to get better is often a 'mask' for other, unconscious wishes. She also noted the discrepancy between the child's inner and outer images of his parents' masculinity and femininity: 'The boy wishes to be immensely big, powerful, rich, sadistic, as in his imagination his father appears to be. The girl wishes to be radiantly beautiful and adored, possessed of unlimited jewels, finery, children, and so on'.[30] She went on to describe the guilt children and adults feel at not realizing their inner sex-typed ideals. She added that in such cases analysis seeks to make conscious the disjunction between inner and outer so as to make more bearable the disappointments and frustrations caused by phantasies of pleasure and retribution.

Freud was outraged. He said that her contribution to the symposium betrayed 'everything we believe of analysis', adding that her criticisms of his daughter were symptomatic of her general 'tendency towards aggression'.[31] Jones now took Joan's side. He maintained that it was entirely consistent with psychoanalysis to insist, as she had done, on the disjunction between the parents' outer behaviour and the child's inner idealizing superego ideas about them. The superego, he argued, is not only formed in response to 'external oppression, threats, etc.', it is also formed in defence against inner feelings, including the 'intolerable distress induced by the non-gratification of various wishes which *in the nature of things* cannot be gratified, e.g. cannibalistic wishes, etc. etc.'[32] Freud replied by applauding Joan's style while also continuing to dismiss her thesis which, like that of Klein, he said, overrated frustration and phantasy to the neglect of other causes of guilt and neurosis.[33]

The next year, however, he warmly greeted her decision to write something of her own. 'Anything you write about yourself personally', he wrote in September 1928, 'is sure of my interest'.[34] The result was 'Womanliness as a masquerade'. Having already spoken about masculinity and femininity in her contribution to the symposium of May 1927, she now drew attention to the dynamic between outer sex-typed display and inner fear of rage and retribution. To illustrate this she described a patient whose greatest sexual pleasure came from masturbating while looking at himself in the mirror wearing a bow tie with his hair parted like that of his sister. In both sexes, she argued, outer adoption of the attributes of either sex may be used as means of warding off inner fear of attack from parents for having 'stolen' these attributes from them.

To illustrate the point further she described women who combine professional work with being wives and mothers, just as she did. She described women seeking to ward off attack by others for their success in male occupations by flirting to win men's reassuring approval, and to prove themselves feminine and therefore innocent of stealing men's traits. A case in point, she said, was an American patient whose father, like Joan's, had been a literary figure and then become involved in politics. Consciously her patient was very rivalrous with, and superior in her attitude to, the father figures she courted in her work and in giving lectures, just as Joan was superior in her attitude to Freud and Jones. She went on to describe how analysis revealed that the patient equated giving lectures with being masculine, for which she sought to avert men's hostility by flirting with them after each of her lectures was over. She also had a dream in which people donned masks to protect themselves from a high tower on a hill being pushed over and falling on them.

To this example Riviere added more general observations regarding Klein's account of babies feeling deprived on being weaned and excluded from their parents' love-making, and of this deprivation leading toddlers to want to retaliate by biting and eating up the mother and the father's penis inside her. She concluded that her American patient wanted to repair the damage she imagined she had done as a child to her mother by using her masculinity to benefit her mother and other women. But this was only on condition that the women she benefited were grateful to her and acknowledged her superiority (just as Riviere assumed women acknowledged hers). It was this condition, Riviere suggested, that made her American patient's task of appeasing and repairing the damage she felt she had done the women in her life so much more endless and exhausting than repairing the damage she felt she had done to men. Most of all, Riviere reported, her patient suffered from her need for supremacy which, when it was disturbed by her analysis, was followed by her becoming anxious, furious and abjectly depressed.

Riviere ended this case history with a general account of the distinction between true and false, inner and outer, femininity. She called true inner femininity 'primary' and said it originates in the pleasure of taking in the mother's milk in breastfeeding, and continues in the pleasure of taking in the man's penis in sex. But it was to other outer displays that she turned in her next essays. They dwelt on jealousy as well as femininity.

Femininity and jealousy

Riviere followed 'Womanliness as a masquerade' with a brief essay about dancing, a subject in which she became actively involved as a member of the Camargo Society. Following Diaghilev's death in August 1929, the society was formed to further British ballet against the claim that ballet was an essentially foreign – especially Russian – art form.[35] Riviere's essay concerned a story told her by a patient about her four-year-old daughter. Following the recent birth of her brother the little girl repeatedly played a game in which she and her mother first had to eat pretend food – bacon, bread, fish. After doing this she would get down from the table with the words, 'Now I must make them grow on the plates again', whereupon she performed an elaborate dance round and round the table, declaring the food they had eaten to be magically restored and 'grown again'. Riviere's account of this story was published in 1930.[36]

That year Riviere was elected a training analyst and member of the Training Committee of the London Institute of Psycho-Analysis.

Among her first trainee analyst patients were John Bowlby (from 1929 to 1933), who later criticized her for focusing too much on the inner world to the neglect of outer reality,[37] and Donald Winnicott (from 1933 to 1938), who likened being in analysis with her to surfacing and seeing the surrounding territory after years of being deep in a ditch. But, like Bowlby, he too later complained that she did not sufficiently emphasize the outer world in attending to what goes on within.[38]

In fact, however, Riviere always insisted on the dynamic between the outer and the inner. In a talk she gave in April 1932 to the British Psycho-Analytical Society,[39] for instance, she drew attention to the way jealousy can act dynamically to outwardly mask inward envy. Freud and Jones had claimed that jealousy – or at least sexual jealousy – is an effect of projecting the wish to be sexually unfaithful outward on to others of whom one then feels jealous. By contrast Riviere claimed that outwardly directed jealousy may serve as a cover for inner envy.

To illustrate the point she described a patient who came into analysis for treatment of various inhibitions, including sexual frigidity – symptoms similar to those for which, according to Jones, she had herself first gone into analysis with him. In analysis, wrote Riviere, her patient became jealously preoccupied with an affair she imagined Riviere was having with her husband. But, said Riviere, this woman's analysis also revealed that her jealousy stemmed from her inwardly empty hunger as a baby, which then drove her enviously to want to rob her mother of everything good inside her which she then equated with milk, faeces and her father's penis. The idea of thus robbing, emptying and ruining her mother was exacerbated by her mother indeed having been ruined, emotionally at least, by a number of disastrous losses – akin perhaps to the losses Riviere's mother also suffered in losing her first son within hours of his birth, and in losing all confidence in her second son making a success of his life. As for Riviere's patient, she sought to reassure herself that her phantasy of robbing her mother had not ruined her by testing it out on other women. She did this by attempting to rob them of their men, but whenever this was likely to succeed she became intensely anxious lest the envy impelling her quest should become obvious. She masked her envy by inverting it – jealously accusing others, Riviere included, of doing the robbing, of robbing her of her men.

At the root of envy masked by jealousy, Riviere claimed, is the hunger of the baby for food. Hunger, she said, is more central to women's than to men's psychology. Women's jealousy is accordingly more often driven by, and a mask for, envy. But this can also occur in men. A striking example is Shakespeare's Othello. He jealously focuses on Desdemona's supposed unfaithfulness to him so as to mask his enviously having robbed her father of her. Iago personifies his envy. Or so Riviere maintained.

Riviere's account of envy informed Klein's later work. For the moment, however, Klein was more occupied with writing *The Psycho-Analysis of Children*, which was published in 1932. She prefaced it with thanks to Riviere for supporting her in her work. Riviere further supported Klein in reviewing Freud's *New Introductory Lectures on Psycho-Analysis* (1933). Three years earlier, in *Civilization and its Discontents* (the title of which Riviere had suggested, and about which she had spoken to the British Psycho-Analytical Society on 5 March 1930), Freud had acknowledged the anger and aggression contributing to children's ferocious inner superego image of their parents. But now, Riviere complained, he overlooked children's aggressive phantasies of eating their parents and how these contribute to their harsh inner image of them. She also complained that he focused too much on external factors – on women's penis envy, for instance – to the neglect of internal figures, including those that are good and are enriched for women, she said, by the pleasure of taking into themselves a lover in sex.[40] But in her next major essay, Riviere wrote more about the inner world as a place of often outwardly masked despair.

Unmasking inner despair

Riviere took as the starting-point for this essay, published in 1936, Freud's description of what he called 'the negative therapeutic reaction', namely the paradoxical worsening of the patient's ills on beginning to get better. Freud attributed this reaction to self-punishment out of guilt about sex. Riviere, by contrast, argued that the negative therapeutic reaction is constituted by outer control, contempt and denial of any value in what the analyst says or does. It serves, she wrote, as an organized mask or defence against the patient's inner relations with those with whom he or she is most involved. Since this mask is an organized defence, piecemeal interpretation is of little use, for in this state of mind women and men are determined to maintain the status quo. They refuse to change. They reject any improvement or praise – just as she rejected praise from Freud in her analysis with him.

Klein's daughter, Melitta Schmideberg, attributed such stasis to fear lest change should lead to something worse. Quoting Schmideberg, Riviere argued that, in the negative therapeutic reaction, the change the patient most fears is revelation of an inner situation of total destruction and collapse. Movingly describing this situation, perhaps on the basis of her own experience, she wrote of it as a world in which

> all one's loved ones *within* are dead and destroyed, all goodness is dispersed, lost, in fragments, wasted and scattered to the winds; nothing is left *within* but utter desolation. Love brings sorrow, and sorrow brings guilt; the intolerable tension mounts, there is no escape, one is utterly alone, there is no one to share or help. Love must die because love is dead. Besides, there would be no one to feed one, and no one whom one could feed, and no food in the world. And more, there would still be magic power in the undying persecutors who can never be exterminated – the ghosts. Death would instantaneously ensue – and one would choose to die by one's own hand before such a position could be realized. (emphasis in original)[41]

Retaining what she called only the 'slenderest belief' in having any capacity to repair this dead and dying inner world, patients in this state of mind feel that anything they try to do about it is a mere fobbing off of desolation. Nevertheless they seek analysis in the belief that it alone dares venture to the fringes of their despair. They cling to analysis. But they also have no hope of it doing any good. Unconsciously they seek to use analysis to stave off death and disintegration. Unconsciously they also seek to reverse and repair the damage they have done within them to those they love. But they resist being told of their goodness in this respect because it makes them despair that this effort will ever amount to anything. They despair of ever making better those they inwardly love. They suspect the analyst's attempt to help them as seducing them away from the burden of restoring their inner world. They worry about also damaging, draining and ruining the analyst. Were they to get well, they would have to use all their energy in never-ending toil to make alive and well those they recall in their minds – figures they not only love but also hate. It is their preoccupation with these inwardly loved and hated figures that makes such patients appear so narcissistically self-preoccupied.

 Their treatment, Riviere concluded, depends on unearthing and bringing to the surface their love – including their good and positive feelings for the analyst. Only thus can the analyst help build up their ability and confidence in having the goodness and love within them that is needed to restore those they feel they have inwardly hated and damaged. But, she insisted, this does not mean the analyst should become the patient's 'ego ideal', as Freud implied.[42] For this is simply to reinforce, through identification with the analyst, the patient's self-idealizing mask against knowing about his or her inner depression and desolation. She warned analysts against being duped by women's and men's false outward show and thus failing to recognize their love and hate for those they recall inwardly. However intense and hard to bear these feelings may be, she said, it is the analyst's task to expose them from under the patient's mask of narcissism and control.

Savagery and love

Arguably Riviere's insights about outer control masking inner desolation came, at least in part, from her own experience of masking with outward haughtiness the desolation wrought in her inner world by the way in which she often snobbishly savaged and dismissed others. Perhaps it was her experience of her own 'harshness', as Paula Heimann described it,[43] and her experience of her own sharp tongue that contributed to her emphasizing the origins of envy in biting phantasies. She spoke more about our earliest phantasies – of biting, gnawing and devouring – on 5 May 1936, in a contribution to the exchange lectures that Ernest Jones organized in an attempt to heal the growing rift between psychoanalysts in London and Vienna.

In her talk, given in Vienna the day before Freud's eightieth birthday, Riviere spoke of babies responding to acute hunger with 'screaming, twitching, twisting, kicking, convulsive breathing, evacuations'.[44] Babies, she said, also discharge their anxieties in the form of phantasies.

> Limbs shall trample, kick and hit; lips, fingers and hands shall suck, twist, pinch; teeth shall bite, gnaw, mangle and cut; mouth shall devour, swallow and 'kill' (annihilate); yes kill by a look, pierce and penetrate; breath and mouth hurt by noise, as the child's own sensitive ears have experienced.[45]

Babies seek to get rid of these phantasies into the mother. They experience her, not themselves, as devouring and devoured bits and pieces. But in also loving the mother as whole and good, she added, the baby feels held together by her. He wants to take her in as a good figure to counteract bad figures inside. This gives rise to phantasies of 'reparation', a concept she now introduced into the Kleinian canon. The baby, she wrote, feels impelled to rescue, repair, restore and preserve good conditions and feelings within him. He also feels impelled to do good to others outside.

Riviere had also given a lecture, along with one by Klein, in London in March 1936, about the infantile origins of good and bad, and of savagery and love. This material was published in 1937 as a book *Love, Hate and Reparation: Two Lectures by Melanie Klein and Joan Riviere*. In her lecture Riviere reminded her audience of the outer evidence of aggression and its pervasiveness. It could be seen in the then prevailing international situation, in 'behaviour in any nursery' and in the 'savage satisfaction, or at least the glee, felt by someone making a cutting retort', which 'can often be seen in his eyes'.[46] She spoke of the curious mixture of love and hate in the baby, of how

> when he is tortured with desire or anger, with uncontrollable, suffocating screaming, and painful, burning evacuations, the whole of his world is one of suffering; it is scalded, torn and racked too. . . . It is our first experience of something like death, a recognition of the non-existence of something, of an overwhelming loss, both in ourselves and in others, as it seems. And this experience brings an awareness of love (in the form of need), at the same moment as, and inextricably bound up with, feelings and uncontrollable sensations of pain and threatened destruction within and without.[47]

These images remain inside us, she said, as a source of our adult hate, aggression, envy, jealousy and greed. Or we see the evil in others, in 'foreigners, or capitalists, or perhaps prostitutes, or a specially hated race'.[48] Alternatively we displace painful figures and feelings on to things. She illustrated the point with the example of the ageing woman (which she herself was now becoming), displacing on to her clothes her image of herself as hopeless and deadly, worn out and ugly, inducing her husband to buy her new ones.

Externalizing what is bad within, she added, involves hate being 'turned outward instead of love'.[49] Or we flee love and goodness in ourselves and seek to preserve and acclaim 'goodness unharmed elsewhere'.[50] But this, she said, makes us greedy, rivalrous and envious – of what is good and loved in the opposite sex, for instance. It also contributes to jealousy which, impelled by the fear of losing those we love, can prevent them from proving us lovable to ourselves. Fleeing from inner to outer reality, she concluded, is to risk entirely replacing one with the other. Inner goodness becomes starved by preoccupation with outer wealth. Conscience, she grieved, was no longer the fashion. Morality had become 'provincial'.

Provincial or not, Riviere was now morally appalled by what she described as a 'really shocking' attack on Klein by her daughter, Melitta, in a talk in March 1937 to the British Psycho-Analytical Society. Riviere's own involvement in the society was now decreasing. At the end of 1937 she resigned as translating editor to the *International Journal of Psycho-Analysis* to devote herself to her clinical work and to doing her own writing. This included a review of Freud's *Auto-biographical Study*, in which she traced the shift from his early concern with outer events – with sexual abuse or 'seduction' – to the inner reality of his patients' phantasies and dreams.[51] Following his death in September 1939, she wrote a tribute to him, appreciating his freedom from all outward 'pose . . . deception or disingenuousness' in attending to the inner wellspring of our behaviour.[52]

But it was Riviere's account of the baby's early phantasies, of how 'Limbs shall trample, kick and hit', that was often quoted thereafter, not least in the British Psycho-Analytical Society's wartime discussions. She herself said little in these debates, apart from a brief intervention on 16 February 1944, noting the baby's dread that, if it cannot get the breast, it will die. In June that year she wrote to Klein's sometime analysand and child analysis supervisee Clifford Scott, lamenting the lack of published writing about Klein's insight into the psychological centrality of what she called the 'conflict between things outside & inside' (underlining in original).[53]

Riviere's own supervisees at this time included Marion Milner, who later recalled Riviere as having told her, 'If you don't do what I say what's the good of your coming!' and that, as 'rather a grand lady', she had snobbishly insisted about her husband, Evelyn, 'Oh, no, he wasn't at Balliol, he was at The House', meaning the Etonian college, Christ Church.[54] Her other wartime supervisees included Herbert Rosenfeld, Henri Rey and Hanna Segal. Segal remembers conversations with Riviere about the work of Conrad, Henry James and Apollinaire, particularly his poem 'Cortège (Moi qui connais les autres)'.[55]

Riviere's theoretical contributions now included noting the phantasy of savagely forcing oneself into others so as to control and possess them. She talked of how this can lead to fear of others retaliating, expressed in fear of burglars, spiders, invasion in war and claustrophobia. Klein quoted this observation in 1946, announcing her theory of projective identification (p. 25 above). And Riviere spoke more about it in 1948, in an (unpublished) talk to the British Psycho-Analytical Society. Her only immediate postwar publications concerned women's reaction to being bereaved or otherwise losing their husbands. She wrote that a woman's grief at this outward loss is compounded by the concomitant loss of the reassurance of being inwardly loved and good.[56] Poignantly her own husband, Evelyn, who had been ill early in their marriage, died of cancer that February. Two years later, in 1947, her mother died, aged ninety-three. Riviere herself was growing old. In her final work she turned to literature to illustrate her previous claims regarding women's and men's inner reality.

Final literary illustrations

In 1948, in a review of Freud's *The Question of Lay Analysis*, Riviere commended his literary style in penetrating and overthrowing his readers' preconceptions and prejudices.[57] Introducing a collection published in 1952 to celebrate Klein's seventieth birthday, she similarly commended Klein's writing. In particular she praised Klein's insights in exploring the unconscious mind's 'deepest recesses' and in going beyond the outward behaviour of babies to reveal that they have an inner life which scientists had hitherto often overlooked but which 'gifted intuitive mothers and women who nurse children have always taken for granted'.[58]

In another essay of 1952 Riviere continued her previous work of exposing our tendency to mask from ourselves our inner world. She attributed this to fear that our inner world might contain nothing but nightmare figures, like the judgemental inner anti-sex superego described by Freud. But, she pointed out, we also preserve in our minds images of those we love, particularly when faced with their loss. She highlighted the point by quoting the following, attributed to a poet called Hoskins:

> By absence this good means I gain,
> That I can catch her,
> Where no one can watch her,
> In some close corner of my brain;
> There I embrace and kiss her,
> And so enjoy her, and none miss her.[59]

The baby, Riviere added, similarly imagines taking in his loved and loving mother so as never to be without her. As adults, she said, we also retain in our minds those we love in order to counteract a fear of losing them, a fear that hatred and aggression might damage or drive them away. It is for this reason, she wrote, quoting Wordsworth, that we cultivate 'that *inward eye* which is the bliss of solitude' (emphasis in original).[60] We comfort ourselves with memories of those we have loved. Or as another poet, Samuel Rogers, put it, also writing of solitude:

> At moments which he calls his own,
> Then, never less alone than when alone,
> Those whom he loved so long and sees no more,
> Loved and still loves – not dead, but gone before –
> He gathers around him.[61]

She also quoted Robert Louis Stevenson comforting himself with the inner image of his dead grandfather as someone who, he wrote, 'moves in my blood, and whispers words to me, and sits efficient in the very knot and centre of my being'.[62]

To highlight inner hell and desolation Riviere cited Dante's *Inferno* and T. S. Eliot's *The Wasteland*. She also wrote of ways in which we make others both the outward repository of our projected image of ourselves and at the same time harbour them within us as both loved and hated, sacred and profane. In Conrad's novel *Arrow of Gold*, for example, the main character tells his long-lost beloved on her return:

> When I have you before my eyes there is such a projection of my whole being towards you that I fail to see you distinctly. I never saw you distinctly till after we had parted. . . . Then you took body in my imagination and my mind seized on a definite form of you for all its adorations – for its profanations too.[63]

In her very last essay, however, Riviere returned once again to ways in which we mask our inner world from ourselves and others. This time she illustrated the point in terms of the hostility that initially greeted Henrik Ibsen's *The Master Builder*. She attributed this to his readers and audience not wanting to know about the inner world the play depicts: its central character, Solness, is plagued by the memory of a fire long ago destroying his family home and of using the insurance proceeds to enlarge his business by taking over that of another builder and his son; the fire also destroyed his wife's happiness and led to the deaths of their children. As she was grief-stricken and despairing, her milk dried up, so the twin sons died of starvation. Solness experiences his wife as a figure who is not so much grieving and dead as persecuting. Having projected his guilt about the fire into her, he experiences her as berating and judging him for infidelities he has in fact never committed. And he feels tyrannized by the builder and son he bought out and whom he now employs in his firm. Above all he finds himself in thrall to a young girl, Hilda, who returns from his past as a demon bent on enslaving and flattering him into giving up his reparative work of building new homes in place of the one destroyed by fire. Instead she incites him to build a tower and climb to the top of it and crown it with a wreath.[64]

Although she produced no more full-length essays, in 1958 Riviere wrote a brief eulogy to Freud. She remembered him urging her to write, saying 'Get it out, produce it, make something of it – *outside you*' (emphasis in original).[65] She likened Freud to an architect 'building up for us in his writings a picture of this world which is unknown to us', a world which, she said, is otherwise masked by our '*not* seeing and *not* knowing' what is within (emphasis in original).[66] She also wrote of her analysis with Freud, alluding to his letters of many years earlier that had drawn attention to her resistance to praise, triumph and success.

Her resistance continued. She refused to have any praise or presents from the British Psycho-Analytical Society on her seventy-fifth birthday. Instead she asked for a party. At it she told an anecdote about her childhood, when her mother would ask her to entertain the guests, whereupon she would get them to watch her paint. But her enthusiasm for winning others' attention through outward show was now nearly over. Earlier that year her first analyst, Ernest Jones, had died, on 11 February 1958. The next year she moved from 4 Stanhope Terrace, where she had lived and worked since the 1930s, to 199 Sussex Gardens. Her friendship with Klein had cooled. She told Bowlby she had no place in Klein's circle of followers in the 1950s.[67] She did, however, go into supervision with one of them, Herbert Rosenfeld, to learn about developments in Kleinian technique.[68] Klein died in 1960 and less than two years later Riviere herself died, on 20 May 1962. She had left orders for the residue of her estate to be left to the Melanie Klein Trust, for no funeral or flowers, and for any donations to be sent to the fund then being collected to keep in England Leonardo's cartoon for the *Virgin and Child with St Anne and the Infant St John*.

Speakers at a meeting of the British Psycho-Analytical Society held in her memory on 3 October 1962 spoke of her 'striving after beauty'.[69] Hanna Segal remembers her originality.[70] In particular her originality lay in her tenaciously going beyond the deceptions of outward beauty, display and control – including the outer displays of femininity and masculinity – to reveal what is inward – particularly our inner world's fears and anxieties, its savagery and desolation. By contrast, as discussed in the next chapter, her fellow Kleinian Adrian Stokes was more outward-looking.

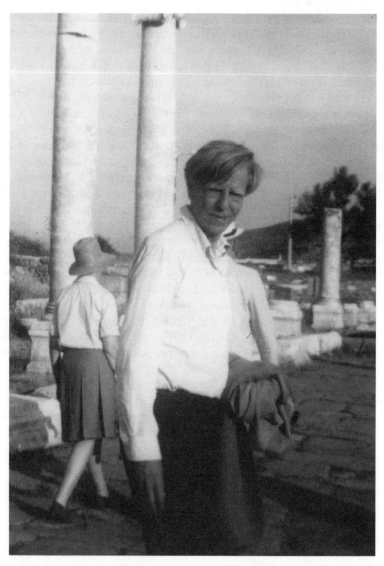

Adrian Stokes in Pergamum, Turkey, 1959/60

4 Adrian Stokes: Ballet and Art

Adrian Stokes was not only more outward-looking than Joan Riviere, he was also outside the Bloomsbury circle. Indeed he loathed it.[1] Nor was he a psychoanalyst. He was an art critic who also wrote about ballet. In doing so he crucially advanced psychoanalytic aesthetics. Whereas Freud and his immediate successors analysed art as expressing unconscious inner phantasy, Adrian Stokes innovatively explored its inner–outer dynamic. In the first place he explored its value as an outwardly light and stable counterpoint to what is often dark and unstable psychologically within us; he had first-hand experience of this through the death of his oldest brother, Philip, during the First World War.

Youthful darkness to light[2]

His brother's death is a recurring theme in Adrian's account of his early years. Philip was four years older than him. Then came Geoffrey, followed by Adrian, who was born on 27 October 1902 at 18 Radnor Place, Bayswater, London. Their father, Durham, was a successful stockbroker from the Midlands who, in 1904, stood as Stepney's Liberal and Labour candidate for Parliament. He supported the cricket club in his country home in Pangbourne, Berkshire. And in the late 1920s he wrote a brief book – in which *inter alia* he argued for the 'subordination of individual consciousness to the spirit of the beehive'.[3] Adrian's widow Ann remembers Durham fondly as amusing but also as a terrible stickler for punctuality and as thrifty to the verge of meanness – refusing to pay for good lighting.

Ann remembers Adrian's mother, Ethel, much more favourably – as tall, beautiful, slim with tiny feet, and as never getting over the death of Philip about whom she talked a lot with Ann. Adrian too was very fond of his mother and, from boarding school onwards, wrote to her every Sunday until her death in 1951. On the other hand he always resented her having betrayed him as a small boy: she had said he could leave boarding school if he did not like it, then sent him to Heddon Court in Cockfosters, Hertfordshire, when he was eight – and abandoned him there, despite his telling her he loathed it.

But in his autobiographical book, *Inside Out* (1947), he wrote neither of her nor of his father. Instead he started it with the dark pall cast over his early life by Philip's death. 'Going down the hill one morning towards Lancaster Gate', he begins, 'my eldest brother remarked on an orange cloud in a dark sky: a thundercloud, he said. And sure enough, that afternoon there was a thunderstorm. . . . a menace that came to violent fruition'.[4] The menace took the shape of a succession of threatening governesses, beginning with a Miss Drew, who came when Adrian was three. He recalled her as a 'very strict . . . and most patriotic Irish lady', who ruled that if shoelaces came undone when they were out walking in Kensington Gardens there would be neither jam nor cake for tea. Dismissed when he was six for mistreating Adrian, Miss Drew was succeeded by Miss Harley. Adrian remembered her as a 'morbidly religious middle-aged woman'. He linked her in his mind with Hyde Park as the 'sum of earlier desolations',[5] with the crashing of his Edwardian world, and with the hymn 'Time like an ever-rolling stream, bears all her sons away'.[6] Intimations of sons and brothers being borne away by war were also signalled for him in 1911 by the coronation of George V, which brought the army to the park; 'red meant soldiers', he wrote, 'angry flowers'.[7] By then Miss Harley had been followed by a French-speaking governess, Mathilde, from Switzerland.

Soon after that, Adrian started day school. He was seven. Images of horrid governesses were succeeded by fears and dangers of being sent away to board:

Under the blare of King's Cross almost every boy is led by a parent far along the platform to be sick, sick from frightened anticipation, in front of the train that will throng him on an iron journey. London drags out along the route; against the will it begins to thin: less and less people live here as if a curse lay on the glowering land. In the semi-country at Barnet we stamp our way over a bridge that clatters; we take brake for the school. Masters are with us, a matron awaits. There will be a fire-practice tomorrow.[8]

He recalled similar alarm and despondency on the journey taking him in 1915 to public school, Rugby, where Philip was headboy. Here Adrian boarded in G. F. Bradby's house. He excelled in sport, particularly tennis. But then, in 1917, Philip, who had been called up the previous year, was killed by a sniper in France. He was nineteen. Adrian was devastated. A fellow pupil at Rugby, William Robson Scott, introduced him to Freud's work. Adrian also took refuge from what he called his 'imaginative despair' in history;[9] he also wrote articles for the school magazine, and was bold enough to send Conrad an essay praising *The Secret Agent* (1907).

After leaving Rugby in 1919, Adrian took up a scholarship in history the next year at Magdalen College, Oxford, but soon transferred to studying philosophy, politics and economics, during which time he contributed an essay to the *Oxford Fortnightly Review* touching on the dualistic philosophies of Immanuel Kant on phenomena and noumena, and of F. H. Bradley on appearance and reality.[10] A fellow student, Eddie Sackville-West, described him then as shy and withdrawn. But he later depicted him – in a novel, *The Ruin*, which he dedicated to Adrian – as an emotional adventurer determined to have complete ascendancy over others. In *Inside Out* Adrian recalled how as a student, travelling on New Year's Day 1922 to Rapallo (where his parents spent the winter), he was transformed on emerging from the Cenis railway tunnel from the dark of northern Europe into the light of Italy:

> the sun shone, the sky was a deep, deep, bold blue. . . . the pure note of the guard's horn . . . sustained and reinforced the process by which time was here laid out as ever-present space. . . . a revealing of things . . . happening entirely outside me . . . [so that] I could not then fear . . . for what might be hidden inside.[11]

The light again and again drew him to Italy. So did the houses and streets, and the old farm buildings, vineyards and olive terraces of Tuscany and the Veneto. But after graduating in 1923 with a second-class degree, he worked as a journalist in London until his father paid for him to travel round the world. He left on 25 August 1923 on the SS *City of Lucknow* for Bombay. While in India in the last months of that year he contributed articles to the Calcutta paper *The Englishman*, about the Taj Mahal and about India's towns, poverty and mysticism. He then travelled east through Burma, Penang, Singapore, Hong Kong, Shanghai, Canada and the USA, where he became completely broke. His father sent him just enough money to pay his fare home: 'So he played his swanny whistle in a band', his widow Ann recalls, 'to buy food on the journey'. Back in England he again worked as a journalist, writing articles about London society, politics and sport, and reviewing books about travel, science and art.

Soon, however, he returned to Italy. In the winter of 1924 he met Osbert Sitwell in Rapallo and had an affair with him. They stayed in Amalfi in late 1925,[12] and in the spring of 1926 travelled together in Spain and Portugal. Osbert modelled the main character in his novel *The Man Who Lost Himself* (1929) in part on Adrian, whom Margaret Gardner later recalled from those days as 'the most fabulous-looking man I think I have ever met. He had fair hair, wonderful large eyes set at a strange sweeping angle, very blue. He looked down most of the time, but when he looked up it was absolutely breath-taking'.[13]

In 1925 Stokes's first book, *The Thread of Ariadne*, was published. It incorporated his Oxford and India articles; in his introduction John Middleton Murry enthused about its central question of 'how to reconcile in one's own living life Interdependence and the Great Commonplaces'.[14] Adrian also began his best-known work – on the Italian Renaissance – in the mid-1920s. Osbert Sitwell persuaded Adrian's father to fund him. At this time, it seems from Adrian's diary of summer 1925, his research was influenced by John Ruskin.[15] It was also influenced by his first visit, on 5 July 1925, to the Tempio Malatestiano in Rimini, where, in the late 1920s, he met Bernard Berenson and despised him for parading the Tempio's treasures to a rich, bored woman tourist. The Tempio was a revelation to him, but it was with a discussion of Giorgione's painting of the *Virgin and Child with Two Saints* that he began his next book, *Sunrise in the West*.[16] The picture hangs over the altar in the cathedral of Castelfranco, north of Venice where, in the mid-1920s, Adrian spent a winter alone, not talking to anyone, immersed in the writings of Gabriele D'Annunzio. He structured *Sunrise in the West* in terms of A. C. Bradley's dualistic philosophy of poetry and prose. In it he also mentioned D. H. Lawrence, whom he met in 1927–8 in Lawrence's home near La Spezia, and whose manuscript of *Lady Chatterley's Lover* he collected in weekly instalments and read overnight before taking it to Lawrence's publisher in Florence.

But the major influence on his work at this time was Ezra Pound, to whom he was introduced in 1926 as already a 'has-been' by a Mr Rhode who invited them to play tennis in Rapallo. Pound in turn recommended Adrian to T. S. Eliot, who was then working for Faber editing *The Criterion*, to which Adrian contributed an article in October 1929 drawing on Pound's *Malatesta Cantos* of 1923–8. They dwell on the Italian warlord Sigismondo Malatesta, who commissioned the building of the Tempio to celebrate his love for a woman called Isotta. A transformation of the Gothic church of San Francesco, the Tempio includes sculptures by Agostino di Duccio, and became a major landmark of the Renaissance in being one of the first buildings to incorporate a Roman triumphal arch in its façade.

Stokes found the Tempio Malatestiano altogether inspiring. But he was still depressed. Worried too perhaps by his bisexuality, he chanced to meet again his fellow Rugbeian Robson Scott, who had just translated Freud's *The Future of an Illusion*. He asked him about psychoanalysis and, after discussing the subject with him for weeks, decided to go into analysis himself. Through Ernest Jones he met Melanie Klein, who agreed to take him on from January 1930. As his analysis got under way he became immensely productive in writing about architecture, sculpture, ballet and painting.

Architecture and sculpture

In an article on Pisanello, published in 1930, Stokes wrote about how the humanism of fifteenth-century Europe made what was inward outward. It made men 'manifest their colour', he wrote, 'embody the soul . . . clear as the midday light'.[17] This drive, he maintained, was particularly well realized by Sigismondo Malatesta, who in the Tempio objectified his energy 'sudden like a glimpse, firm like a flower in full bloom . . . instant manifestation . . . mass all at once like mountains in unbroken sunlight'.[18] Taking issue with the assertion of Walter Pater that all art approximates to music, which achieves its effect over time, Stokes celebrated the Tempio for its immediately present outwardness.

In his next book, *The Quattro Cento*, published in 1932, Stokes again emphasized this factor as contributing to all that is best in architecture and sculpture. He deplored the usually celebrated achievements of the Renaissance – those of the Florentines Brunelleschi, Ghiberti, Luca della Robbia and others – as either too aggressive and 'gouged out' or too repressed and reserved. Much better, he wrote, were the early Renaissance marble carvings in Florence and Verona, and the architecture and sculpture of the Palazzo Ducale in Urbino and of the Tempio in Rimini in achieving what he called all at once outward opening, unifying, full flowering, blossoming.

But his analysis kept him in London and away from Italy. He warned Pound – whom, it turned out, he saw only twice again, and then only fleetingly in 1935 and 1938 – 'I shan't be in Italy for years'.[19] One of his homes in London was a flat near the

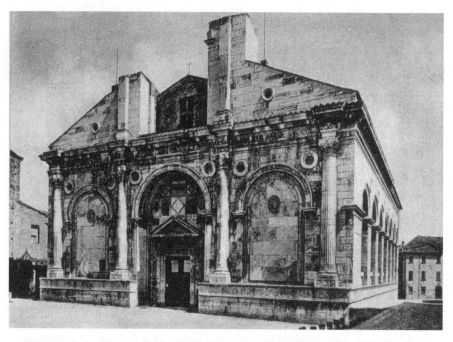

Façade of the Tempio Malatestiano, Rimini, designed by Leon Battista
Alberti

Embankment Gardens, in the eighteenth-century Adelphi terrace, designed by the Adam brothers. In 1933 he reviewed Klein's *The Psycho-Analysis of Children*,[20] and began formulating what was to become his major aesthetic tenet, which he later cast in Kleinian terms, distinguishing between outwardly-dominated carving and inwardly-dominated modelling.

Carving, he wrote, focuses on what is outside while modelling focuses on what is inside. Modelling involves the artist imposing on his medium what is within him. In another article of 1933 (written for *The Spectator* while its regular art critic, Anthony Blunt, was away), he illustrated the distinction with the paintings and collages of his friend Ben Nicholson. He likened what he termed their carving quality to farming, which brings forth from the earth what is already good and fruitful within it. By contrast he likened modelling to manufacture, which involves the transmuting of raw materials according to the manufacturer's will.[21]

In 1934 Stokes moved to the recently built avant-garde Isokon flats, designed by Wells Coates, in Lawn Road, Hampstead. Other residents included the Bauhaus architects Marcel Breuer and Walter Gropius, the sculptor Henry Moore and the artist László Moholy-Nagy.[22] That year Stokes's book *Stones of Rimini* was published; he dedicated it to the painter Mollie Higgins (with whom he travelled in Yugoslavia, and who later married the psychoanalyst Gilbert Debenham). Carving, he insisted, manifests the essence of life. It throws 'an inner ferment outward into definite art and thought'. Modelling, by contrast, 'is not uncovered but created': 'The modeller *realizes* his design with clay. Unlike the carver, he does not envisage that conception as enclosed in his raw material' (emphasis in original).[23]

He began *Stones of Rimini* announcing 'I write of stone'.[24] He went on to detail ways in which the sculptor Agostino di Duccio used stone to externalize what was within it. He described how, in the bas-reliefs he carved for the Tempio, Agostino made the formation of marble from water flowing over shells outwardly manifest. Marble, he wrote, lends itself particularly well to this externalizing process because of its translucence, its diffuse light and the polishing, rounding and layering involved in its carving. Agostino's mastery of perspective enabled him to reveal, graduate, flatten and relate each surface to the next. His figures thereby issue from the stone. Stokes likened them to 'flowers that thrust and open their faces to the sun'.[25]

Furthermore, by replacing Christian figures such as Christ and the Virgin Mary with classical figures such as Diana and Mercury, Agostino translated into outward form the inner ideas of fecundity and trade that these figures symbolize and represent. He also

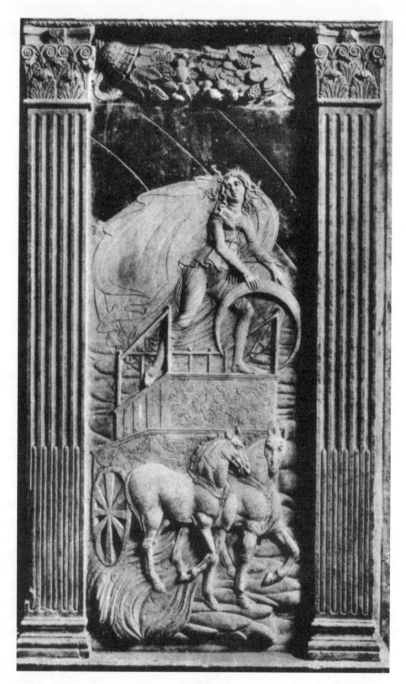

Diana

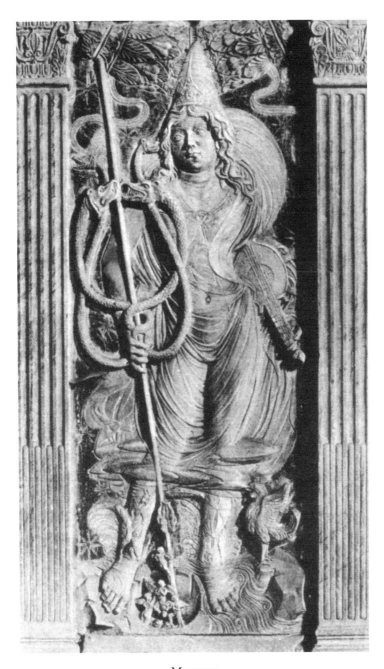

Mercury

rendered the inner fluidity from which marble is made in carving them in which their 'draperies open and close like the rhythmic washing to and fro of tresses of seaweed clothing a far rock beneath clear water . . . drawn up by a spring tide, by the curious influence of Diana . . . resurrected as the sods are upturned by the process she has set in motion'.[26] Similarly, wrote Stokes, Alberti used classical motifs to transform the Tempio's Gothic façade into 'stone-blossom' and 'incrustation'. The result, he said, conveys 'organic connexion between architectural members and between background and ornament' with the façade's pilasters looking as if they had 'grown from the wall-space . . . steadfastly like a flower'. (see p. 74)[27]

Stokes had initially intended to write more about Agostino and Alberti in a book to complete a trilogy with *The Quattro Cento* and *Stones of Rimini*, but he abandoned the project, perhaps because it was inspired by Pound with whose Fascist sympathies he became increasingly uneasy.[28] Perhaps too he abandoned it because his continuing analysis with Klein reduced the homoerotic fantasies of domination underlying his interest in the warlord Sigismondo, whose life and love the Tempio celebrates.[29] Whatever the reason, his next books were about ballet.

Ballet

Adrian had been introduced to ballet by the Sitwells, and, with the death of Diaghilev in 1929, when the Russian ballet was in danger of collapse, he offered all the money he had – £300 – to the ballet's London impresario, Eric Wollheim, to help save it. 'Give what you like, my boy', his father told him, 'but you won't get another penny from *me*'. But Wollheim rejected the offer from Adrian, who instead supported the ballet by writing in its praise, beginning with his infectiously enthusiastic book *To-Night the Ballet* (1934).

Unlike many of his other books which are often off-puttingly enigmatic and obscure, *To-Night the Ballet* is a masterpiece of lucidity not only about dance but about art generally as outward consummation of what he called 'inner ferment . . . in the form of display'.[30] Ballet, he insisted, manifests 'dreams in the flesh, an inner world on an illuminated stage . . . an inner world externalized with all the insistence and the verve of which the outer world is capable'.[31] The ballerina, he claimed, 'shows us the deepest emotions as something theatrical or outward and self-contained'.[32] This is especially the case in classical ballet, so much does its technique involve the dancer 'turning out' to reveal 'as much of himself as possible to the spectator'.[33]

In 1935 Adrian's brother Geoffrey died after suffering for many years from some kind of sleeping sickness associated with his involvement in the Battle of Jutland during the First World War. In his second ballet book, *Russian Ballets* (1935), in contrast to what has been called his rather 'clogged'[34] writing about art, Stokes both lauded the outward effect of ballet and conveyed this effect through making the reader see outwardly, as though before his very eyes, each of the ballet performances described.

Starting with *La boutique fantasque*, he showed how an inner world is made manifest through toys in a toyshop coming alive. Of *Swan Lake* he wrote: 'It would, indeed, be irreconcilable with balletic poetry should the dancer *imitate* a swan. She *is* the swan in human form: additional grace and power is added to the bird' (emphasis in original).[35] He went on to describe how the waywardness of a dream is made into a consistent image by a dancer in *Les Sylphides*; how a son's vision of gaining his potency is realized in *The Firebird*; how a couple's inward anxiety is rendered outward in *Les présages*; and how the heroic attitude of Hermes in *Choreartium* transforms Brahms's music from hearing into seeing. The book ends with a comparison of the externalization achieved in *Choreartium* to that of Piero della Francesca, who 'painting the grievous theme of Christ's flagellation, made the figure of Christ more column-shaped than the column to which he is tied, translated the ignoble scene, without loss of its poignancy, to appear no less contained than an episode from Homer in the hall of an Aegean palace'.[36] In his next book, *Colour and Form*, he focused altogether on painting.

Painting

Colour and Form was published in 1937. A couple of years before Stokes had himself become a painter with the help of a painter friend, Adrian Kent. He began with landscapes in Cornwall, to which he was attracted because his brother Philip had enjoyed studying the geology there. In 1936 he met another painter, Margaret Mellis, whom he later married. She was twenty-one, and he met her at a Cézanne exhibition in Paris on his way to the south of France, where he spent 1936–7 in a villa in Sanary, in which Aldous Huxley also sometimes stayed. On returning to London he moved into a top-floor flat a few doors away from an art school at 12 Fitzroy Street, which had just been started by Claude Rogers, Victor Pasmore and William Coldstream (who, like Ben Nicholson, had also attended Stokes's prep school Heddon Court). In February 1938 the art school moved to Euston Road and came to be known as the Euston

Road school. Its associates included Graham Bell, Lawrence Gowing, Rodrigo Moynihan and Stephen Spender.[37] In March 1937 Stokes reviewed an exhibition of Ben Nicholson's work at the Lefèvre Galleries, which he commended along with abstract art generally in so far as its texture or gradations of colour enable what he called subjective 'fantasies of inner disorder' to achieve calm 'objective harmony'.[38]

Colour and Form begins in a similar vein. He argued that outer space affords 'wished-for certainty and freedom' from the disorder of loving and hateful figures within.[39] Painting achieves this effect, he claimed, through 'identity-in-difference', a term he took from the philosopher F. H. Bradley. It is achieved, he wrote, not through the elusive otherness of 'shiny surfaces',[40] but through the luminosity of inner or self-lit – 'as if breathing'[41] – matt surface colours rendering each and every form equally and immediately present. He illustrated the point with the example of Picasso's *Woman with a Mandoline*. Its addition and substraction of colour, he wrote, stabilizes the otherwise unpeaceful, mixed-up, inner archetypal figures bequeathed to us from childhood. Self-lit colour, he noted, is particularly evident in objects seen in evening light: in the frescoes of Piero della Francesca; and in the carrying through of a theme by Giorgione who, with his phrase *'per una sola occhiata'* ('through a single glance'), affirmed painting above sculpture in immediately communicating its subject.[42]

Stokes also praised Pieter Bruegel the elder, particularly his *Fall of Icarus*, and its emphasis that outward life continues whatever the fate of individuals within it. He lauded the painting's interrelation of colour and form: the background peasant with his blue shirt 'shaped from his folded arms' mirroring 'the blue from the green-blue milky sea, whitened and fleeced from association with his sheep';[43] the foreground figure, with his plough, 'belonging in very substance to that earth which he symbolically carved to greater fruitfulness', his shape springing out from the 'total insistence of all the landscape'.[44] It was a painting which W. H. Auden, whom Stokes had first met in the early 1930s, also celebrated in his poem 'Musée des Beaux Arts'.[45]

In 1938 Stokes's own paintings, along with those of Ivor Hitchens and others, were exhibited at the Lefèvre Galleries. Stokes later painted several still-lifes of bottles, illuminating the inside-out theme to which he often returned in his writings. In 1938, too, Stokes's analysis with Klein ended; he also designed a poster with Margaret Mellis for an anti-Franco demonstration in Trafalgar Square in May and married Margaret in June. The next year, with the outbreak of war, the couple moved to Cornwall.

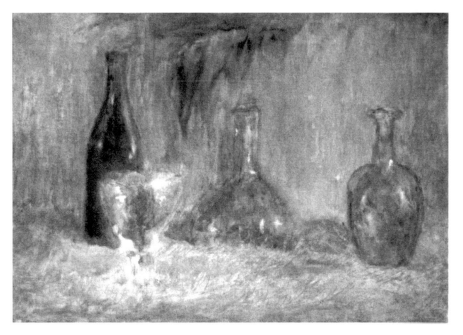

Adrian Stokes, *Still-life*, 1965

Continuing inside out

After the war Stokes was to attend to what is inward in art, but for the moment he continued to focus in his writing on art's outwardness. He was offered – but declined – the post of curator of the National Gallery on its evacuation to Wales. Instead he contributed to the war effort by joining the Home Guard and setting up a market garden in Little Park Owles, Carbis Bay, Cornwall. Ben Nicholson, Barbara Hepworth and their triplets came to stay in 1939. So did the honeymooning Spenders. In 1940 Naum Gabo moved to the area. And in May of that year Margaret's seventeen-year-old sister, Ann, came to stay, a few months before the birth of Adrian's and Margaret's son, Telfer, on 3 October 1940. Adrian encouraged his sister-in-law to do ballet; this took her in June 1941 to London, where she joined the WRNS. Meanwhile, Adrian became involved in looking after a fisherman, Alfred Wallis, whose naive paintings he had commended in *Colour and Form*. When Wallis died in August 1942 Adrian took care of his estate.

Stokes's next book, *Venice*, published in 1945, again focused on the outwardness of art. He detailed Venice's architecture to illustrate what he called the 'intoxication' of the early Italian Renaissance with 'showing outer form . . . stabilizing an inner content as outer shape'.[46] He felt this process to be epitomized in Giorgione's controversial painting *The Tempest*, of which he wrote: 'every clearly seen object appears to possess equal importance, equal insistence whatever the size, owing to the inter-locking palpability of local colour'.[47] He also discussed the threat posed to Venice by the war and the 'godlessness' of the external world. He urged his readers to find goodness within. It stems, he now argued (perhaps influenced by his son's recent birth), from the baby's early experience of taking in his mother as a good and separate figure outside him.

Also in 1945, Stokes published the first of several articles for the *International Journal of Psycho-Analysis*, 'Concerning art and metapsychology', in which he quoted Freud in advancing his own long-held view of art as 'transposing to the external world a formless inner nexus'.[48] This theme is reiterated in *Inside Out* (dedicated to his wife), in which he also returned to the topic of early mothering. The heart of human nature, he now wrote, is to be found in the nursery, in the suffering for example of a seventeen-month-old girl miserably crying, 'Mum, mum, mum, mum, mum'.[49] He went on to quote Joan Riviere's insistence on our inner need to love and be loved. He added that, like the child determined to put together what he imagines tearing apart inside, the artist similarly takes apart and puts things together outside.[50]

Stokes's next book, *Cézanne*, was published in 1947. He commended the outwardness of evenly distributed colour and form in Cézanne's paintings of bathers, and of a landscape near Aix-en-Provence he wrote: 'the surfaces and images of surfaces are so distinct and incisive . . . enhanced by the mosaic of the field behind upon the hill, by the pyramids of red roof by the sprouting conical foliage of the trees'.[51]

By this time Adrian's marriage was in difficulties. He left Margaret in Cornwall, returned to London, went into analysis again with Klein (from 1946 to 1947), and began courting his sister-in-law, Ann. Having divorced Margaret, he pressed Ann to marry him, to which she finally agreed, generously encouraged, she says, by Margaret, and with the blessing of their father – a minister of the Church of Scotland in Edinburgh – who quipped that the marriage had better work since he had no more daughters. But it was against British law to marry a sister-in-law, so Adrian and Ann went abroad and on 22 May 1947 they married in Ascona, near Locarno, in Ticino in Italian Switzerland. It was here that their first child, called Philip after Adrian's brother, was born on 18 February 1948.

Adrian's next book, *Art and Science*, was published the following year. He dedicated it to Ann. In it he continued to affirm the outwardness of art, this time in terms of the use made by Alberti, Piero and Giorgione of the fifteenth-century sciences of architecture and perspective, and their use of tone in unifying surfaces in pursuit of what Adrian had long called the 'emblematic' – meaning the process by which an inner state is objectified and externalized.

Outside in

Written in Ascona in 1948–9, and initially called *Outside In*, but renamed *Smooth and Rough* on its publication in 1951, Adrian's next book (also dedicated to Ann) turns from what is external to what is within. In April 1950 the devaluation of the franc had led him and Ann to move from Switzerland back to England to live in a house called Heathgate, in Buckleberry, Berkshire. In early 1951 there was an exhibition of Adrian's work at the Leger Galleries, and that year he also published further articles about ballet and about Piero della Francesca.[52] His and Ann's second child, Ariadne, was born in Reading on 10 June 1951, and in the autumn they moved to Hurtwood House, Albury, near Guildford.

Not long afterwards they moved again. Ariadne was diagnosed as schizophrenic (and later as brain-damaged). When she was three she began analysis four times a week with Esther Bick in West Hampstead, and the family moved in 1952 to nearby Church Row in Hampstead. From there Philip started going to prep school at The Hall, and Ariadne went to school in Fitzjohn's Avenue. Ann describes her daughter at this time as 'an enchanting, fairy-like tiny child with funny, fluttering movements with her arms at half stretch followed by a jump as if across a puddle and turn round to flutter again before another jump . . . the fluttering so exactly like Adrian's own hand movements when deep in thought that even Philip remarked on it'.[53]

Adrian still wrote for Faber and *The Spectator*.[54] Perhaps influenced by Ariadne's treatment, he now distinguished between modelling and carving in terms of Klein's concept of the schizoid mechanism of projective identification (see p. 25), whereby we put figures from within us into others, thus experiencing them not noly as outside but the same as what is within us. His increasing Kleinianism led many in the art world – including Kenneth Clark and Geoffrey Faber, who had once declared Stokes to be the greatest prose-writer of his generation – to become disenchanted with his work.

His books were now mostly published by Tavistock, beginning with *Michelangelo* in 1955. In it he dwelt on the deaths that Michelangelo endured: his mother died when he was six, followed by the deaths of his younger brother and of his father. Stokes drew attention to how Michelangelo imagined them as inner figures in his mind. 'My brother is painted on my memory', Michaelangelo wrote, 'but you, father, are sculpted alive in the middle of my heart'.[55] Stokes went on to describe Michelangelo's drive to repair depressing loss and destruction of external figures within. Looking at his sculpture, we become witnesses to this outer–inner process, to what Stokes described as

> a heroic, constant movement that overcomes, or rather absorbs, depression and the state of being overpowered. . . . Whatever the ferment, she [the Michelangelesque woman] must possess the brooding calm of a fine youth, the marble brow, the generous, unsullied resignation . . . *Night* and *Dawn* in the Medici chapel . . . [find] the hidden depressive centre in ourselves . . . an eloquence of substances that is read by the tactile element inseparable from vision, by the wordless Braille of undimmed eyes.[56]

In his essay 'Form in art' (1955), Stokes similarly depicted Rembrandt conveying a 'benign and unifying experience' through bringing together outer and inner, visual and muscular apprehension of his sitters' characters with his use of pictorial texture and shape.[57] After mentioning Marion Milner's account of the baby experiencing himself and his mother as 'breast and mouth . . . fused into one',[58] the essay ends with Klein's account of babies integrating the splitting of their outer and inner world through internalizing the mother as good and loved.

Stokes initially presented this and other essays to the Imago Group, which he had co-founded with the composer Robert Still for fellow analysands to pursue the non-clinical applications of psychoanalysis. The group's members and visitors included Stuart Hampshire, the LSE philosopher J. O. Wisdom, Marion Milner, Wilfred Bion, Hanna Segal, Donald Meltzer, Anton Ehrenzweig and Roger Money-Kyrle and his wife (who apparently slept from beginning to end of every meeting). It met monthly from 1954 (until its disbandment in 1972), often in the Portland Mews house of Ernest Jones's widow, Kathaerine.

Several of Adrian's contributions were later collected and put together by the film critic and psychoanalyst Eric Rhode (the son of the man who first introduced him to Pound in 1926).[59] From 1956 he often published in the *International Journal of Psycho-Analysis* and also wrote for *Encounter*, beginning in March that year with a review of Rudolph Arnheim's book *Art and Visual Perception*.[60] For the next couple of years, he isolated himself from almost everyone except his family. Perhaps he was drawing on his own experience when he wrote that the artist, like the child, is inwardly destroyed and seeks to repair what he tears apart. In 1958 he described how artists enable their public to share in this destructive-reparative process, as he believed Monet did in his paintings:

> The colour, as well as the brush-strokes and the surfaces represented, was apt to appear in fragments so as to allow of a generous reconstruction in the name of light . . . generous in the sense that you can see the artist at work, you can see how he reconstitutes surprisingly the dominant effect, puts on the paint.[61]

In his final work, however, Stokes attended not only to outer–inner destruction and repair but also to the peace and repose afforded by art and ballet as they outwardly envelop us within.

Enveloping outer–inner repose

Stokes came to this more restful view of art after meeting Richard Wollheim (the son of Eric Wollheim) at the Royal Academy's exhibition *The Age of Louis XIV*, held in 1958. Perhaps this restful view also came from his being happier in his marriage to Ann than he had ever been before. He wrote now of the goodness of mothers bringing about inner repose. In *Greek Culture and the Ego* (1958), he wrote that the 'good enveloping inner object is the crux of the well-integrated ego',[62] and that its peace and integration stem from the baby, once inside the mother, experiencing her as outwardly enveloping him within.

In October 1960 Stokes was made a Trustee of the Tate Gallery, a post he kept until retiring in 1967 (when he refused a knighthood, perhaps to prevent realization of Sitwell's prediction, in his 1929 novel about him, that he would be decorated). During the 1960s he went on writing, notably an article on architecture,[63] and a book, published in 1961, called *Three Essays on the Painting of Our Time*, in which he argued: 'The great work of art is surrounded by silence. It remains palpably "out there" yet none the less enwraps us; we do not so much absorb as become ourselves absorbed.'[64] To illustrate art's outer–inner 'is-ness' (a term he borrowed from Aldous Huxley), he quoted Van Gogh writing to his brother, 'Beyond the head . . . I paint infinity, I make a plain background of the richest, intensest blue . . . and by this simple combination . . . I get a mysterious effect, like a star in the depth of the azure sky'.[65] Art, he insisted, is '*par excellence* a self-sufficient object as well as a configuration that we absorb'.[66] He wrote further of this dual outer–inner aspect of art in commending Coldstream's paintings for meeting our 'desire for undictated stillness in ourselves, [as well as] for stable people and things in the outside world'.[67] Enjoying art involves contemplation and resignation.[68]

Resignation, however, was not his attitude to the threatened destruction of Venice by failure to protect it from flooding, against which he protested with others in a letter to *The Times* (published on 18 December 1962). By then he had become increasingly friendly with Richard Wollheim, who had begun analysis with the Kleinian Lesley Sohn, and who called in on Stokes once or twice a week after seeing Sohn. Wollheim described Stokes as also something of an analyst – sitting with his back to him, half-listening but with the 'most total concentration upon the person that I have ever observed'.[69] His thoughts flew off at tangents. But he was also firm, particularly in defending psychoanalysis. He talked about art, exhibitions and friends – more about the present than the past.

It was the same in Stokes's writing. Dedicating *Painting and the Inner World* (1963) to his son Telfer (who had graduated from the Slade and was now studying at Brooklyn Museum Art School), Stokes again stressed immediacy in the visual arts. To this he now added his perception of art embracing us within, as in Turner's later paintings, of which he wrote: 'humidity is sucked from water, the core of fire from flame, leaving an iridescence through which we witness an object's ceremonious identity: whereupon space and light envelop them and us . . . whirlpool of fire and water . . . beneficence in space'.[70]

Stokes's own painting and writing were now approaching their end, but this last phase of his work was very productive. He went on to write reviews of Klein's *Our Adult World and Other Essays*,[71] Segal's *Introduction to the Work of Melanie Klein*,[72] a book about French monastic architecture,[73] an article about Herbert Read[74] and an account of his and Ann's postwar years in Switzerland.[75] On 17 November 1964 he was interviewed by Leonie Cohn on the BBC Third Programme about Klein's work. Two months later he had an exhibition with Lawrence Gowing at the Marlborough Fine Art gallery,[76] for which he was interviewed for the *Arts Review*.[77] On 12 August 1965 the *Times Literary Supplement* carried a letter praising his work, with eighteen distinguished signatories.

In 1965 Stokes also published two more books: one about Venice, illustrated by John Piper;[78] the other, *The Invitation in Art*,[79] in which he dwelt on art's compelling incantation to draw us in, to identify with and become enveloped by it, while also remaining detached in its contemplation. In a talk to the Imago Group on 6 July 1965 he referred to this process as 'being taken out of one's self'.[80] In *Michelangelo* (1955), he had maintained that art involves inner fusion and external 'out-thereness'. Now he reworked the theme in the *British Journal of Aesthetics*.[81] He used the resulting article as the conclusion to his last book, *Reflections on the Nude* (1967), comparing Michelangelo's statue of *Day* (in the Medici Chapel of San Lorenzo, Florence) with the effect achieved by dancers in classical ballet in overriding inner restlessness and strain with outer density and calm.[82]

In December 1968 there was another exhibition at the Marlborough Fine Art gallery of his paintings (together with those of Keith Vaughan). His articles of the late 1960s and early 1970s include one about Ben Nicholson[83] and a few book reviews.[84] In his last full-length article, using material which he had presented in lectures to art students in Camberwell and Chelsea, he again wrote, as he had at the beginning of *Painting and the Inner World*, of art's enveloping inner–outer effect: 'The artist is the furniture removal man of great ambition, converting vague objects from the dark into chair and dresser laid on the street, insisting upon neighbourhood communion, the inner with the outer'.[85]

But he was finding it increasingly difficult to sustain the concentration needed for such writing.[86] Or perhaps he had written everything he had to say of any urgency in prose.[87] Instead he increasingly wrote poetry, including the following to his mentally ill daughter Ariadne:

> Hugging yourself to preserve a skin
>   That barely separates
>   Barely resists the air;
> Stiff-jointed, bent, muscle-stretched
> Day and night against unintegration[88]

He likened her tragedy in not being securely integrated and enveloped from outside in to being a 'sack of potatoes . . . speckled with tears and holes'.

Ariadne was now sixteen. She refused to continue her analysis with Esther Bick. Having long coped with her at home, Adrian began to be persuaded she should live elsewhere.[89] Eventually she went to live in a retreat house run by nuns near Haywards Heath, West Sussex. For the moment, as things were difficult between her and her parents, her doctors advised they should see her less often. This contributed to their going away, in 1969, on a cruise around Greece.

Soon after that Adrian became ill with cancer. In 1971 he had a colostomy, and seemed to recover well. So much so that he and Ann went on another Greek cruise. But on their return he started losing his memory. He could not add up or put his papers in order. Scans revealed cancer in his brain and his chest. This did not prevent him from celebrating his seventieth birthday that October. But two days after finishing his last painting, he died on 15 December 1972.

Shortly thereafter, on 28 December, *The Listener* published two of his poems in his memory, including one addressing the integration of inner and outer, past and present:

> You are the animal I love
> You interweave belonging there and then
>   Patient fretted pattern
>   On ambiguous mesh
>   In presence of the flesh.[90]

In February to March 1973 the Tate devoted an exhibition to Stokes's paintings. Wollheim described them as often of 'bottles, landscapes, and occasionally nudes aimed at stillness'.[91] But it is above all the emphasis in his writing on the enveloping inward outwardness and inside-out aspects of ballet and art that has endured.[92] So too does the clinical work of his near contemporary, the psychoanalyst Herbert Rosenfeld, in treating the ill-effects of this inner–outer process going awry.

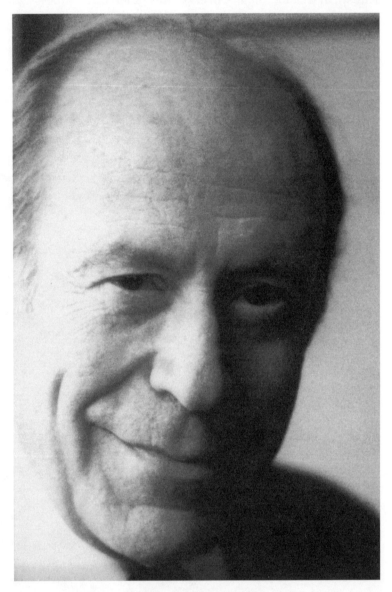

Herbert Rosenfeld, *c.*1980

5   Herbert Rosenfeld: Schizophrenics and Gangsters

Herbert Rosenfeld was remarkable in being one of the first psycho-analytsts to extend Freud's talking cure method to treating schizo-phrenics. In doing so he used Klein's insights about children's phantasies of intruding, getting into and wreaking havoc in their mothers' bodies, and their terror of their mothers similarly getting into and wreaking havoc in them. He also used the discoveries of Riviere and Klein regarding fears of becoming claustrophobically imprisoned in others. Drawing on what he learnt from talking with schizophrenic patients, Rosenfeld pioneered recognition of the fears of less ill patients of their outer behaviour being driven by gangster-like figures within them.

Rosenfeld arguably drew on a related inner–outer dynamic that drove him to spend almost no time with his immediate family, but hours with others outside it, particularly with the women and men he treated. His devotion to his patients resulted in a wealth of clini-cal detail, as discussed below. On the other hand, because he was rather unforthcoming (at least in print) about himself, it is difficult to establish much about his personal life beyond psychoanalysis.

Outsiders[1]

The few known facts include his birth in Nuremberg on 2 July 1910, two years after the birth of his oldest sister Edith; two more sisters were born after him, Marion when he was nearly four, and Inge when he was nearly eight. Their mother, Lili, was twelve years younger than their father Arthur, and is remembered by her grandchildren as very warm-hearted. She had a predilection for mysticism and, when her children were young, was attracted to the ideas of Johannes Müller – a priest turned philosopher and quasi-guru founder of a retreat centre at Schloss Elmau, near Germany's Bavarian border with Austria, where the family often went on holiday.

Herbert himself distrusted mysticism. He preferred a more outward, scientific attitude to life. He also gained a reputation in the family for liking to talk with outsiders – strangers, for instance, whom he happened to meet at Germany's annual carnivals and fairs. Preferring psychology to becoming involved in the hop merchant business that his father ran with his uncle Kurd, he decided, with his father's support, to study medicine at Munich University. He later wrote of being disappointed in the psychology he learnt as an undergraduate, as it focused on outward behaviour to the neglect of what goes on inwardly. He was also disappointed in his professor, Oswald Bumke, who had an anti-Freudian, Kraepelinian approach to psychiatry. Later he too warned against Freud, at least against interpreting too quickly the patient's sexual feelings about the analyst. For, he said, it can result in the patient feeling sexually intruded into and assaulted, as happened with one of Rosenfeld's Munich patients: her condition deteriorated after he said that her hearing voices telling her she would soon get married meant she was sexually attracted to him.

Whatever his resulting reservations about talking too soon with patients about sex, Rosenfeld followed Freud in being committed to treating patients by talking with them. But after Hitler's rise to power in 1933, Jews were debarred from much professional work. Rosenfeld managed to continue direct work with patients only through the help of one of his professors, a man called Benjamin, who ran a small private hospital, Kindersheim, near Munich. The hospital specialized in treating psychologically disturbed children. Working with them Rosenfeld was able to complete his MD thesis, 'Multiple absences in childhood'. He graduated in 1934, but by the end of that year Benjamin was no longer running Kindersheim and Rosenfeld had to go elsewhere for clinical experience.

So he left Germany, and in 1935 got a post in London at Guy's Hospital, where he attended R. D. Gillespie's psychodynamically oriented lectures. After completing the year's practice needed to take his final qualifying exams, he went in January 1936 to study for them in Edinburgh. Here he worked in the city's Royal Infirmary and, after taking the exams that autumn, returned to London and worked in Hammersmith Hospital. But again he was stopped from seeing patients, this time by a ruling that doctors from overseas could work in England only if they were experienced or specialists. His residence permit was cancelled and he was offered work in either Australia or India.

By then, however, he had met his future wife, the nineteen-year-old Lottie Kupfer. Born in Frankfurt, she had completed her last years of schooling in Hampstead. Having previously wanted to become a musician, she was now training as a physiotherapist. Her parents had settled in England. Soon, after selling the family business, Rosenfeld's parents had settled in London – at 23 Brim Hill, East Finchley. Herbert now discovered that he too could stay if he registered as a psychotherapy student at the Tavistock Clinic (then evacuated from Malet Place in Bloomsbury to Hampstead). He accordingly applied and, while waiting to start its two-year training course in autumn 1937, worked as a locum in the mental hospital at Littlemore, near Oxford.

Here he was again discouraged from seeing patients. He was told he need see them for only an hour and a half a day, that the rest of the day was his own. But he was determined to spend more time with patients and selected for psychotherapy a patient he called Edgar who, apart from bouts of catatonia and violence, was friendly and told Rosenfeld he suffered electric shocks on going to bed at night. Rosenfeld explained that they were sexual feelings about which, it seems, Edgar was previously ignorant. Grateful for Rosenfeld's help, he became less frightened and more co-operative on the ward. When Rosenfeld returned to the hospital some months later, he found Edgar's improvement had led to his being discharged, his improvement being attributed by the physician superintendent in charge not to Rosenfeld's help but to spontaneous remission.

Meanwhile Rosenfeld had been working for a couple of months at the Maudsley Hospital in south-east London. Here too his psychiatric colleagues downplayed the value of talking with schizophrenic patients, since, they claimed, their problems were biologiclly not psychologically determined. But Rosenfeld persisted. He talked with a sixteen-year-old, Eliza, whose symptoms included experiencing sexual feelings inside as though they came from outside, from her mother whom she violently attacked on first learning in early adolescence that, as she put it, she had been born through a hole in her mother's body. But Rosenfeld was not allowed to treat Eliza. He was, however, allowed to treat another patient, Edward, who improved and was discharged. When Edward broke down again a couple of years later, he remembered Rosenfeld's help and asked his father to arrange for him to see him again in therapy, which he did and, after six months of seeing Rosenfeld twice weekly, Edward was well enough to return to teaching at the boarding school where he had been a pupil seven years before.

By then Rosenfeld had completed his Tavistock training, during which he also went into analysis with an analyst from Berlin. But he found it unhelpful in so far as it focused on inner Oedipal and castration conflicts to the neglect of their outward transference on to the analyst. Meanwhile his own patients included a man called Thomas, who was troubled by obsessional ideas, but when it became clear that Thomas was schizophrenic, Rosenfeld's Tavistock teachers persuaded him to have him referred for hospital treatment. Thomas wrote from hospital saying how abandoned he felt. Determined not to similarly abandon others, Rosenfeld soon after agreed to take on a private patient referred to him by one of his Tavistock colleagues, Dr Bevan-Brown. The patient was thirty-five and had first broken down ten years before, when he became convinced his mother wanted to teach him sex by having intercourse with him. With Rosenfeld's help he recovered sufficiently to hold down a job as a caretaker in a psychiatric nursing home, make friends and, on retiring, live with his sister.

At the end of his Tavistock training, Rosenfeld went into treatment with a second analyst, whom he found much more helpful than the first in addressing his transference feelings about him. But with the outbreak of war the analyst was called up. Being an enemy alien disqualified Rosenfeld from military service, and he stayed in London. A year after he had completed his Tavistock training, he and Lottie married, on 25 February 1941, and moved into a flat in Vernon Court, Hendon Way.

Lottie was then in analysis with Paula Heimann. Rosenfeld found that Lottie's account of her treatment helped him in treating his own patients. When he heard that Melanie Klein, from whom Heimann had learnt her approach, was returning from evacuation in Pitlochry to London, he applied and was taken on for analysis by her. In May 1942 he applied for psychoanalytic training, which began in July. His and Lottie's first child, Robert, was born on 27 January 1943. The following January Rosenfeld took on his first training patient under the supervision of Susan Isaacs, and then a second training patient, called Mildred.

Mildred[2]

Rosenfeld's account of Mildred's case was the first published case history of an adult suffering a schizophrenic breakdown treated according to Klein's theories. Initially Mildred's treatment, like that of Rosenfeld's other early schizophrenic patients, seemed likely to founder. When it became clear that Mildred might become ill with schizophrenia, Rosenfeld's supervisor, Sylvia Payne, urged him to stop the analysis. But Rosenfeld was determined not to abandon Mildred as he had his Tavistock patient, Thomas. He persuaded Payne to agree to his continuing to treat Mildred in which he was helped, he said, by Klein enabling him to know about his own tendency towards schizophrenically splitting off and putting feelings from himself into others. Riviere had described this as involving fear of becoming claustrophobically imprisoned in others, a notion adopted by Klein in her concept of projective identification (see p. 25 above). Rosenfeld in turn applied this concept clinically. In a talk to the British Psycho-Analytical Society on 5 March 1947 he spoke of Mildred's fear of becoming imprisoned in others.

This fear was not immediately apparent, and indeed Mildred initially complained of having no fears or feelings, and of almost total withdrawal from others, a withdrawal that had first begun when, aged nineteen months, she had reacted to her brother's birth by stopping talking. She was less withdrawn following her sister's birth four years later and, apart from becoming somewhat paranoid after a couple of operations for mastoiditis when she was eight, she did well and went to boarding school when she was twelve. But after she left, at the age of seventeen, she broke down with one physical ailment after another. This culminated in a period of uncontrollable crying. By 1939 she had recovered sufficiently to work in the Auxiliary Territorial Service, but soon after she started she broke down again. On recovering she joined the Land Army but was invalided out because of continuing physical ills, including suffering flu for several months before first seeing Rosenfeld in his Welbeck Street consulting-room in March 1944.

By then she was twenty-nine. She began treatment feeling so blanketed off from others and deadlocked emotionally that she despaired of ever getting better. Again she had flu. On recovering she told Rosenfeld how much she enjoyed being ill, staying in bed and indulging phantasies of living warm and snug in someone else. She thought it was her mother. Certainly her mother had always said Mildred had not wanted to be born. Now she did not want to get up. That was why she was so often late for her sessions, sometimes arriving only a few minutes before they were due to end. At first she seemed unconcerned about this. But one day she arrived distressed that her mother had given her breakfast in bed but she still could not get up.

She despaired of ever taking in anything good to get her going. Rosenfeld talking with her in these terms led to her telling him another phantasy, one she had entertained since childhood, of a devil attacking good people and keeping them imprisoned and tied up in dungeons, gagged and bound. Whenever they showed signs of moving, the devil attacked and bound them tighter than ever. There was no point fighting him. He was so strong. The only solution was to ignore him.

Mildred similarly ignored herself – her feelings. She split off and denied all good feelings in herself and Rosenfeld, and located them instead in a young relative she scarcely knew. But then she became terrified of being overwhelmed by sadness on learning that the relative had become engaged. So she cut herself off from this feeling too. All that remained were bad feelings of persecution and fear, including such intense fear of Rosenfeld she briefly became schizophrenic. She became convinced he was the same as the imprisoning devil in her phantasy, that he was pushing her into a hole, putting a lid on and leaving her trapped. Everything good had to be kept separate and apart from him lest, like her imagined devil, he take what was good from her, make it bad, or make her feelings about what was good disappear altogether. She became convinced that whatever he said was aimed at stopping her thinking her own thoughts and aimed at getting her to think his thoughts instead. She suffered the delusion that he was an all-powerful figure, bent on getting into her to control and rob her of her very self, against which she withdrew into an all-powerful world of her own.

Only very gradually did Mildred begin to respond to Rosenfeld again as someone distinct and outside her delusions about him. As she did so she said she could not bear coming to see him because it made her feel so hopeless. At this he suggested that perhaps this was because, now she had been in analysis with him for nineteen months, she dreaded he would give up on her just as she felt her mother gave up on her when she was nineteen months old and her brother was born. At this she became slightly more hopeful. But then she wanted to attack Rosenfeld, as she had wanted to attack her mother following her brother's birth. She also reacted, as she had then, by attacking, stopping and cutting herself off from all inner wanting and feeling.

Gradually, through Rosenfeld talking with her about her thus negating her feelings, Mildred began to become aware of them. She brought her feelings together. She became aware of feeling good as well as bad about Rosenfeld, and grateful to him for enabling her to integrate these contrary feelings and experience herself as whole. Soon after she fell deeply in love and got engaged. All went well except for a brief episode when her fiancé had to go abroad for a couple of months. Briefly she again cut herself off from her feelings. At the same time she imagined herself swelling up like a balloon to twelve times her own size, while at the same time also experiencing herself as a tiny figure inside. 'Expectancy', she said, had something to do with it. It transpired that she withdrew whenever she experienced someone outside expecting something from her or forcing themselves into her, just as she imagined forcing herself into others and emptying them – as in the image of the empty balloon – of everything good she expected from them.

It was the same with Rosenfeld: she wanted to force herself into him. But then she dreaded he would force himself into her. It was the same with sex. She dreaded her fiancé forcing his penis into her. Talking with Rosenfeld about this dread, however, led to it diminishing. She became more able to experience and take in his analysis not as something to be dreaded but as good and helpful within her. Similarly with her fiancé. She became less fearful of sex with him, enjoyed it, married, and when his job soon afterwards took them abroad felt able to end her analysis, confident that her marriage would succeed, despite having suffered a brief paranoid schizophrenic breakdown during her analysis. But what of patients whose paranoia is longer-lasting?

Paranoia

In 1911 Freud had described just such a patient in analysing the autobiographical account of 1903 by a Leipzig-born judge, Daniel Paul Schreber, of his schizophrenic breakdowns that began when he was forty-two. These included the delusion that he had a mission to redeem the world, and that to do so he had been transformed into a woman out of whom a new race would be born. He imagined God impregnating him. But he also castigated God as plotting to murder his soul and sexually abuse him. Freud argued that paranoia, in such cases, stems from defending against childhood homosexual desire for the same-sex parent by turning this desire into hatred and projecting it into others of whom the patient then feels the object of their hatred and attack, this justifying him in hating and destroying all feeling for them. Freud likened the resulting catastrophe to that bemoaned by Goethe's Faust, who grieves:

> Woe! Woe!
> Thou hast it destroyed,
> The beautiful world,
> With powerful fist!
> In ruins 'tis hurled.[3]

But why did Schreber break down? Was it perhaps due to the depression caused by his having just been passed over for promotion, and by his becoming middle-aged and still having no children? Certainly Schreber's own account of his case suggests this possibility. Discussing his case, Klein argued that depression – including catastrophic hatred and destruction of all feelings for others – is not so much an effect of paranoia as its cause. Arguably it was to fend off depressing hatred and destruction of others that impelled Schreber to get rid of these hated figures into others; his paranoia might have been derived from his experience of others retaliating by extruding into him the hated figures he extruded into them.

Klein had long treated the effects of this inside-out process in children. It was left to her medically qualified colleagues, however, to pioneer its treatment in adults, as Rosenfeld had in treating not only Mildred, but more chronically paranoid patients. A case in point was a patient described by Rosenfeld in a number of papers,[4] whom he saw in his consulting-room in 36 Woronzow Road, near Primrose Hill, where he and his family moved in 1947.

I will call the patient involved Peter. He was a forty-year-old artist, and had become openly homosexual fifteen years before on learning that homosexuality could be punished under English law. A year later he began living with an older man who looked after him. At the same time he had other homosexual relationships in which he was the more active partner, and after five years began an intense affair, interrupted in 1939 by the war when Peter, who was a pacifist, became a conscientious objector. He worked on the land and enjoyed it, but, towards the end of the war, became increasingly depressed, made a suicide attempt, and in 1946 went into analysis. Three months later, however, his lover returned and he stopped going for analysis. But he soon became disappointed in him, became increasingly promiscuous, painted his face, and enjoyed people decrying him as a prostitute. Enjoyment then turned to paranoia. He began hearing outside voices in his head, abusing and sneering at him for soliciting and being a queen. He shouted at strangers whom he suspected of shouting at him, which resulted in his being hospitalized for three months in the summer of 1947. A leucotomy briefly reduced his paranoia. But then the voices returned and he again sought analysis. Finding that his first analyst could not take him on, he saw Rosenfeld and started treatment with him in March 1948.

In the course of his analysis he told Rosenfeld how, as a small child, he used to want to smear himself with shit, and how, when he was four, he took soot from the chimney and blackened his face with it, just as he painted his face in prostituting himself as a homosexual. He also remembered himself as a child excitedly riding on his father's knee. As he did so he would imagine shitting in his pants without his father knowing. Telling Rosenfeld these memories allayed his depression and anxiety. It was as though, said Rosenfeld, he got rid of these feelings, together with his shit and penis, into him. It freed Peter from depression and left him feeling elated. But elation was soon followed by his again hearing voices, which Rosenfeld explained as being caused by fear that Rosenfeld would force back into him the depressing badness he imagined extruding into him.

Soon, perhaps through Rosenfeld putting this into words, Peter began to get better. When he first saw Rosenfeld he had been completely unable to paint, which he attributed to his previous analyst equating his painting with smearing shit, with what was bad, destructive and depressing. But Rosenfeld pointed out he also felt shit was good. He reminded him how he studied how best to use it in manuring his garden. Through thus talking about what was good, as well as bad, Peter recovered his ability to paint.

Previously he had confused good and bad. The confusion was expressed in a dream in which he imagined several lobsters lying side by side. One of them crept on top of another and completely swallowed it, whereupon it became a horrid skeletal creature. Peter felt sorry for it as though it were the effect of his bad self swallowing his good, loving and sexual self. To get away from this mixed-up, good-bad, inwardly imagined creature he put it out of himself into others – including into someone about whom he complained before telling this dream.

Talking with Rosenfeld about how he thus put into others his inner confusion of good and bad led him increasingly to distinguish between them. In another dream he represented their confusion through imagining that Christmases were all stuck together and that he shook hands with a woman who suffered the same disease as him – schizophrenia. He then dreamt a woman was boiling and mixing old and new stools of shit in a saucepan. The first of these two dreams led him to talk of his parents stuck together with the simple and sexually free people living in their village. He both derided and valued them as good and bad, simple and free. Similarly in dreaming of shaking hands with the schizophrenic woman, he was both good and bad, friendly and hostile in allying himself with her and attributing to her his illness. In the second dream, however, he also faced and distinguished between these feelings – between good and bad, old and new, food and shit. Returning the next day to the first dream, he said that Rosenfeld's interpretations were like Christmas presents. Since he gave them every day, they too were 'stuck together'. He added that it was during the Christmas break following his last analysis that he had become completely mad. But as he increasingly faced good and bad and the distinction between them – between Christmas presents and his madness, for instance – his paranoia about outside attacking voices getting into him decreased.

Rosenfeld described this patient's recovery from paranoia in a talk to his fellow analysts in Zurich in August 1949. Rosenfeld's father died that year, and on 4 March 1949 his wife, Lottie, gave birth to their second child, Angie. Soon afterwards Lottie became ill with TB. To offset any upset this might have caused, Angie she was later sent, aged three, for analysis with Esther Bick. As for Rosenfeld's own patients, they included in 1952 an in-patient, whose case illuminates particularly starkly the inside-out processes Rosenfeld had first detailed in describing his treatment of Mildred's and Peter's paranoia.

In-patient[5]

I will call the patient involved David. He was born abroad in 1930. It was not until he was sixteen, when he threatened to throw himself off the parapet outside the fourth-floor bedroom he was sharing on holiday with his younger brother, that his parents noticed something was wrong with him. Soon after that he accused his father of not telling him the facts of life, fell in love with a ballet dancer and broke down completely when she left him.

Over the next three years he suffered hallucinations, was confused and sometimes violent and was treated with electric shock and ninety insulin coma therapies. The superintendent of the private mental institution where he was hospitalized said he was the worst case of schizophrenia he had ever dealt with – he ranged between being dangerous and impulsive or withdrawn and mute. None of the doctors or nurses could make contact with him. But two of Rosenfeld's colleagues made some headway. They felt David might be accessible to psychoanalysis, and referred him to Rosenfeld, who first saw him in January 1952. By then David was twenty. For a fortnight he was brought by car to see Rosenfeld in his Woronzow Road consulting-room. After that Rosenfeld saw him in the hospital for an hour and twenty minutes every day except Sundays.

Contrary to Freud's claim that schizophrenics are too self-absorbed to be accessible to psychoanalysis, David immediately responded to Rosenfeld's attempt to help him. He began by looking puzzled and confused. Then he said, 'Resurrection'. At this Rosenfeld said, 'Resurrection means to become alive'. 'Are you Jesus?', David asked. Jesus could do miracles, Rosenfeld observed, and added that David hoped he would also do a miracle and make him better. At this David looked distressed and uncertain. He was silent for a long time. Then he mentioned a Dr A, who had treated him with physical methods for over a year. Again he was silent for a long time. Then he said, 'Catholicism'. Rosenfeld explained that he had believed in Dr A and was disappointed his treatment had failed. To this David replied emphatically, 'The Russians *were* our allies'. He felt Dr A was an ally but had turned against him. And David was afraid, Rosenfeld went on, that he too would change from an ally into an enemy. David agreed. 'That is true', he said. Then he became more talkative. He spoke of sexual problems, of circumcision, of a boy who used to sit next to him at school, but the trouble was the boy who sat on the other side. Rosenfeld explained that David began to like him as he liked the boy at school, wanted him to himself, but realized he also had other patients. At this David became restless. He got up saying, 'One must get out at once – I better go now'. Later he mumbled, 'I must have a saw'.

The next day he seemed much more confused and preoccupied with his hallucinations. He took no notice of Rosenfeld. He looked around the room, trying to fix his eyes on one spot after another. Rosenfeld commented that he had lost him and was trying to find him again. 'Not true', David retorted. He continued his search around the room. Rosenfeld noted that he felt he had lost and was looking for himself in his room. At this David looked straight at Rosenfeld and told him, 'One has to find one's own roots'. A little later he added, 'I do not know whether it is right liking you *too* much'. Rosenfeld explained that David was frightened that liking Rosenfeld too much meant getting inside him and losing himself and his roots. David agreed. 'I want to go on peacefully in *my own* way'. He became absolutely still and did not move for the next ten minutes. Then he said there was a heavy burden on his shoulder. Looking at Rosenfeld, he added, 'It is lighter now'. Rosenfeld observed that he wanted to rid himself quickly of his burden.

At their next meeting David was very restless. He laughed a great deal and made movements with his hands as if to brush Rosenfeld away. He wanted to show him the treatment was no good, said Rosenfeld. 'No good at all', David laughed. To this Rosenfeld noted that David had expected a miracle cure, and felt that his ensuing disappointment and anger had destroyed Rosenfeld and made him and his treatment no good. David responded by looking frightened and suspicious. He jumped out of his seat as if Rosenfeld attacked him when he spoke. He felt Rosenfeld did indeed attack him, that he put words into him to muddle him up. That was why he shut himself off from Rosenfeld and tried to take no notice of him. After Rosenfeld explained his shutting himself off in these terms, David became less frightened.

David went on to talk about colours, about Rosenfeld's blue diary being brown. He showed Rosenfeld how, in attacking him, he turned him into the colour of shit as revenge for Rosenfeld putting the muddle – the shit – into him. In later sessions it turned out that the shit was connected with the burden he had mentioned becoming lighter at the end of their second meeting. It became lighter through his shifting the depression and bad feelings in him into Rosenfeld and into countless others outside. But he then felt they attacked him from outside in.

Four weeks into his analysis, David was having tea one day with his father when one of the nurses, Sister X, affectionately put her arms around his shoulders. Dreading her attacking, forcing herself into, and taking possession of him, David reacted by hitting her hard on the forehead. After this he said nothing to Rosenfeld at their next two meetings. At the following meeting he said he had destroyed the whole world. Later he said 'Afraid', repeated the word 'Eli' (meaning 'God') several times, and looked very dejected, his head drooping on his chest.

Rosenfeld explained that on attacking Sister X David felt he had destroyed the whole world. Only Eli could put it right. Still David said nothing. He started talking only when Rosenfeld mentioned guilt and fear of being attacked. 'I can't stand it any more', David responded. He stared at the table saying, 'It is all broadened out, what are all the men going to feel?'. He could not stand the guilt and depression inside, Rosenfeld explained, so he put these feelings outside where they all broadened out between lots of men. He wondered what all these different parts of him in them felt. At this David looked at one of his fingers, which was bent, with the words 'I can't do any more, I can't do it all'. Then he pointed to one of Rosenfeld's fingers, which was also slightly bent, and said, 'I am afraid of this finger'.

Equating his own bent finger with the guilt and depression he felt inside, feeling he could not do any more with these feelings in him, and putting them instead into Rosenfeld and his bent finger, he now became frightened Rosenfeld would put these feelings back into him. Over the next ten days he was so frightened of what might come into him from outside that he stopped eating and drinking. But after Rosenfeld put it to him that he was frightened of taking in good things, as well as bad, lest they make him feel guilty again, he drank a glass of orange juice one of the nurses had left for him on the table.

One Sunday, a fortnight later, he was about to attack one of the nurses when he stopped himself, turned very pale, and said, 'Hiroshima'. The next day he told Rosenfeld, 'You are too late', followed by 'I cannot look', several times adding, 'I can't do anything'. He repeatedly mentioned death. Then he stopped talking. He opened his mouth as if to speak. But no words emerged. He could not speak, Rosenfeld said, for fear of what was inside and might come out. 'Blood', David said. At this Rosenfeld explained that he had missed him over the weekend, felt very impatient, and had killed him in his mind. Now Rosenfeld had arrived it was too late to help. He was frightened to look at the destruction. It felt too real and bloody.

The next day he told Rosenfeld, 'We have to stop, I can't do it any more'. He again showed him his bent finger, mentioned death and blood and shrugged his shoulders. Again Rosenfeld stressed how real his inner attack on him had been, to which David said, 'I want to have shock treatment'. Rosenfeld asked what this meant to him. 'Death', he immediately replied. He felt he should be killed as punishment, said Rosenfeld. David agreed.

This was followed the next day by his giving further evidence of taking into himself the guilt and depression he sought to put into Rosenfeld after his attack on Sister X. He touched Rosenfeld's hand several times and looked at him anxiously. Rosenfeld said he wanted to see if he was all right, at which David echoed him by asking, 'Are you all right?'. He was afraid he had hurt him, said Rosenfeld, to which David replied by saying 'chicken', 'heat' and 'diarrhoea', signifying imagining having eaten Rosenfeld like a chicken, destroying him with diarrhoea, and worry lest he had destroyed him outside.

After explaining this, Rosenfeld found David the next day looking intently in his hand. Rosenfeld asked what he saw. 'Crater', David replied. What was inside? 'Nothing – empty'. He was frightened Rosenfeld was in the crater – dead. Later he closed his hand and squeezed it tight. He was imprisoning and crushing him inside, said Rosenfeld. He replied by continuing to squeeze his hand, looking withdrawn. Then he suddenly got up, turned around frightened, and left the room. When the nurses brought him back Rosenfeld noted that, when he squeezed and imprisoned him in his hand, the room felt it was imprisoning him. He felt he was Rosenfeld. He felt guilty about what he was doing to Rosenfeld in him. Learning in this way about what he was thus doing and feeling, David became less anxious as he returned to squeezing his hand.

The next day, however, he became very frightened when he was out walking with the nurses. He suddenly stopped, stared at the ground and would not go on. When they asked what the matter was, he said he heard voices threatening to kill him and that he had stopped walking because there was an abyss ahead. Eventually he calmed down. Later he fell forward a couple of times, as though dead. Talking about it later, Rosenfeld said that David felt he had killed and destroyed him in the crater and that Rosenfeld was taking revenge. That was why he heard voices threatening to kill him and fell down, as if dead.

At this David became more able to experience figures in his mind not only as vengeful, attacking and attacked, but also as helpful and good. He began the next session looking in his pocket for his handkerchief. He was also looking for the part of himself, said Rosenfeld, which helped control him but which he could not find. He often lost this part of himself because he could not stand the anxiety and guilt. At this he looked straight at Rosenfeld saying, 'The problem is how to feel the fear'. He wanted to feel the fear, and anxiety and guilt inside, Rosenfeld explained, because he realized he needed an inner something or someone to control him. To this he responded by looking out of the window at a man trimming the hedges outside. Rosenfeld pointed out that the man was trimming the hedges to shape and control them without damaging them. David wanted to feel Rosenfeld was similarly helpfully and undamagingly controlling him inside.

After this, and for the first time, he talked rationally with the doctors and nurses for several hours almost every day for the next three weeks – an improvement Rosenfeld attributed to his being more able to acknowledge his need for a helpful controlling figure within him reducing his anxiety about being attacked. He was now more able to face depression and the need to repair the damage he felt inside. He represented this inner situation outwardly in terms of a black box in the corner of the room where he and Rosenfeld met; he repeatedly opened the box to describe the bones inside, which were used to teach the student nurses and doctors anatomy. At about this time he also told one of the nurses he had a great deal to worry about but that it would be all right in the end.

Once he asked Rosenfeld, 'How can I get out of the tomb?' He again felt he had put his depression into him, that he was entombed in him and wanted Rosenfeld's help to get out. Other times he seemed preoccupied with making things better inside himself. When Rosenfeld asked what he was doing, he said he was rebuilding heaven. Sadly, however, his rebuilding and recovery soon stopped. His mother returned from abroad and pressed for him to be treated with physical methods. A leucotomy was suggested. David again became violent and uncontrollable. His analysis with Rosenfeld ended – four months after it had begun – its premature cessation perhaps being somewhat compensated for in so far as his treatment gave Rosenfeld insights he used in treating other patients at home.

Home and away

Among patients Rosenfeld treated at home was a seventeen-year-old, Anne,[6] who had first broken down with auditory and visual hallucinations when she was thirteen. Rosenfeld began treating her in May 1953. At first she came to see him with her mother, whom she also evidently heard as a voice in her head trying to make her look stupid in front of him. Later, on seeing him on her own, Ann evidently both wanted him to get into her and was frightened of it. She represented this, said Rosenfeld, in the way she greedily smoked a cigarette and then turned its burning end towards her lips complaining, as she did so, that she felt sick. Sometimes she was so fearful of his getting into her and of her becoming imprisoned in him that she could not bear to come to see him. He was then able to continue her treatment only by going to see her in her home, where she talked of being in 'somebody else's coat', asked him what he kept under his jacket and put her hand in his pocket. He talked more with her about her thus expressing her wish to get into him (the counterpart of her fear of his getting into her), after which she became less driven to do so. She became less distraught, coped well with the first holiday break in her treatment in August 1953 and was able to deal with the anxieties of returning to continue her treatment in his consulting-room in his Woronzow Road home that September.

Sometimes Rosenfeld saw Anne every day except Sunday. His daughter Angie wonders whether his giving so much time to his patients may have been due to his transferring to psychoanalysis – as did many other analysts at this time – a need for the sense of belonging he had lost on becoming a refugee. Since his death Angie too has become involved in psychoanalysis, as a group analyst. She remembers becoming intrigued by psychoanalysis as a child, when the family had to be silent every fifty minutes as his patients came and went. By then the Rosenfelds had another child, Suzanne, born on 24 March 1954, who, like her mother, Lottie, also became a musician – a viola player.

Throughout his offsprings' childhood Rosenfeld continued to devote almost all his time to psychoanalysis. He saw patients every day except Sundays, often starting before 8 a.m. and seeing them all day – apart from a short break at 1 1, and a nap and a walk with the dog after lunch – until early evening. Then he would often run a seminar for students at home or go out to meetings elsewhere.

In what little time remained he enjoyed reading and going to the opera. Most of all, says Angie, he loved the ballet, *Coppelia* for instance. He loved the music because it wasn't spoken, she explains, 'it was such a rest after all the talking he did with patients'. He also enjoyed art: he bought a Rodin sculpture of intertwined hands; and he collected paintings. He wanted to fill the walls with their richness. Thinking she too had artistic talent, he and Lottie sent her to Adrian Stokes for lessons – of which she had four or five, Adrian impressing her as kind and patient, but as also somewhat frightening on account of his importance and charisma.

Like Stokes, Rosenfeld played tennis. Angie remembers the television being on all day during Wimbledon, and being a ball girl for her father when he played tennis in Regent's Park on Sundays with another psychoanalyst, Frank Phillips. He also played tennis in Angmering-on-Sea, a village near Brighton, where, a couple of years after his mother died in 1961, he and Lottie bought a house for the family to spend weekends, and near which their son Robert, who became a teacher, now lives in East Preston.

Rosenfeld's work often took him to Los Angeles, where he would stay with his younger sister Marion. As one of the first psychoanalysts to bring Klein's ideas to the US, he gave talks there and in Canada about his discoveries concerning schizophrenics' fears of intruding into and being intruded into and imprisoned in others. He also talked about the anxieties of less ill patients of feeling intruded into by gangster-like figures ruling their outward behaviour from within.

Gangsters

Rosenfeld gave several examples of patients complaining of just such gangster-like figures impelling them into addiction or hypochondria.[7] An example was a man whom I will call Joseph, who first came into analysis with Rosenfeld aged twenty-one, complaining of pressure in his chest and a variety of ills in his head, limbs, heart and stomach.[8] Shortly before getting married he dreamt he was walking with his fiancée towards his room. Suddenly a door opened and a man, who had tried to rob the room, came out. Joseph challenged the man and put his hand into his pockets. But he could not find anything he had stolen in them, at which the man smiled. A couple of people were standing nearby; they did nothing to help, even though Joseph shouted. The gangster smiled and got away, leaving Joseph frightened that he would never forgive him for having challenged him, and that he would sooner or later return to wreak vengeance on him, as he figuratively did in the parts of his body with which Joseph was hypochondriacally preoccupied. In analysis, says Rosenfeld, he similarly sought enviously to get into and rob him. Through Rosenfeld talking with him in these terms, however, he was gradually able to experience his analyst not as enviously robbed and emptied but as good and helpful within him, and by July 1960 felt able to end his analysis and remained well.

Generalizing from such patients, Rosenfeld concluded that the imagined gangster figures plaguing them inside are a reaction against hating, feeling dependent on and enviously wanting to rob and spoil love and goodness in others. This impulse, he said, often contributes to what Freud and Riviere called the negative therapeutic reaction (see pp. 54 and 60 above). He claimed that the reason some patients paradoxically react negatively, getting worse just after beginning to get better in analysis, is because they mount a gangster-like self-castigating attack on themselves as pathetically dependent and weak for wanting, needing or using the analyst's help.

Examples of this reaction included a psychotic patient addicted for years to seeing prostitutes once or twice every day.[9] With analysis he became less driven to do so. But just as he began to get better, he heard a voice in his head telling him it would be fine for him to see a prostitute, everything would be all right if he did. Nevertheless, despite this inner voice, and the negative therapeutic reaction to which it led, he continued to get better. But now he sometimes became murderously angry with others, particularly when he felt they were better than him. This led to his becoming obsessed with anxiety in case he indeed inadvertently murdered someone, though gradually his obsession with voices and images of others as so bad he had to murder them diminished. He became more able to own rather than split off his feelings of badness into them.

During the 1960s and 1970s Rosenfeld continued to devote himself to analysing the ills done by these inner–outer processes. His patients included a Hollywood film star famed for acting the part of a real-life gangster. Determined to learn as much as he could about his patients, Rosenfeld asked his nephew Andreas Heyne, in whom he seems to have confided more than in his immediate family, and whose father was an actor, to tell him all he knew about acting – about how actors feel before a première, how they learn a script, everything.

It was the same, writes Andreas, when Rosenfeld had a broker as a patient. He read all the economics journals he could find. Andreas asked him why he did so much research about what his patients did, to which his uncle replied that he did not know but had to find out why they chose the work they did. Perhaps the broker was the businessman patient whom Rosenfeld called Robert and through whose case he provided the most extensive account of the inner gangster-like figures that can rule our lives.

Robert was thirty-seven and unmarried when he came into analysis.[10] As the problems for which he sought treatment diminished, and as his personal relationships and work began to improve, he woke up with panic attacks at night. He felt his hands did not belong to him, that they wanted to destroy something by tearing it up, that he had to give in to them, that they were too powerful for him to control. They seemed to be controlled by someone else – by someone who figured in one of his dreams as a very powerful, arrogant man. He was 9 ft tall, taller even than Rosenfeld, who was 6 ft 1 in (and than Rosenfeld's son, Robert, who was 6 ft 3 ins and after whom Rosenfeld may have unconsciously named this patient in writing about him).

This dream figure insisted he had to be obeyed. Rosenfeld explained him as a divided figure, attacking Robert for depending on his parents as a child and on Rosenfeld in analysis. Robert was surprised by Rosenfeld's interpretation, but it relieved him, and he gradually experienced his hands as more under his own control at night. And he no longer split off, but instead became more aware of his own, very tall-seeming, powerful self. He became consciously arrogant, and openly sneered at Rosenfeld for wasting his time seeing patients all day.

Robert then had another dream, in which he was running a long-distance race while a young woman did everything she could to interfere and mislead him. She had no belief in what he did. Her brother, who was called Mundy, was even more aggressive. He snarled like a wild beast, even at her. Mundy led Robert to think of the Monday sessions he often missed because of the extended weekend business trips he took away. Mundy's sister – the interfering, disbelieving woman – similarly figured in his mind as someone who arrogantly and contemptuously dismissed Rosenfeld's help. As his analysis progressed, however, he became more able to know about, acknowledge, and take in his analysis as helpful, free of these figures ganging up and attacking it. He dreamt of himself as a little girl receiving and appreciating her teacher's help.

Final teaching

Rosenfeld too was a teacher. His teaching in the last decade of his life included speaking about what he had learnt from Robert's analysis in a talk to his fellow analysts in Vienna in 1971. In the 1960s his students had included Lesley Sohn and Donald Meltzer. He used their cases in a talk in Boston in 1964 to illustrate the fears of schizophrenic patients of being imprisoned in, or intruded into by others.[11] During the late 1970s and early 1980s he also taught in France, Germany, Argentina and Italy, often about the inner gangster-like figures who, as with his patient Robert, can attack and stop women and men acknowledging and taking in what is good and helpful from outside. Sometimes, he wrote, these gangsters constitute a veritable Mafia. A case in point was a patient who dreamt of himself as four bandits pinned to the ground by Rosenfeld, who figured in the dream as a policeman against whom the bandits protested that they killed only because they were starving.[12]

Rosenfeld spoke about this patient in a talk in Jersualem in August 1977. By then his and Lottie's children had grown up and left home. In the early 1970s he and Lottie moved to 9 Meadow Bank, in a new housing complex on Primrose Hill Road. He arranged to see patients in a converted garage. But the arrangement was not very satisfactory. Things improved when they moved four years later to Burgess Hill (near their first Vernon Court home on Hendon Way). Here Rosenfeld continued teaching and seeing patients, despite suffering a melanoma on his chest, for which he had a skin graft in 1981, and despite falling over and breaking his leg following a seminar in Munich in 1982. Here he was hospitalized for four months since he also suffered pneumonia following a pulmonary embolism. On recovering he went on working and teaching. This included teaching about women's and men's vulnerability to feeling intruded into by the analyst's verbalizing their gangster-like envious destructiveness of anything good. He mentioned this varying vulnerability, be it thin- or thick-skinned, in a final 'afterthought' to his second and last book, *Impasse and Interpretation*, published posthumously in 1987.

Rosenfeld was completing it in 1986. That November he discussed with Angie, when she was visiting for her daughter's first birthday, plans to reduce his workload and visit India and Australia. The next day, however, after a full day seeing patients, and when a group of qualifying analysts were gathering in an upstairs room for a seminar, he was found collapsed with a stroke at his desk in his study below. Some said the stroke was due to overwork. He rallied, but a few days later he got worse, perhaps because of another stroke. Now he could no longer speak. 'It was awful', says Angie, 'someone whose whole way of being was through talking not being able to say a single word'. Ten days later, on 29 November 1986, he died. He was seventy-six. His illness and his funeral – at Golders Green Crematorium – brought together for the first time his world within his immediate family and many outside it – friends, colleagues, students and patients from Switzerland, America and elsewhere. Their coming from far afield was well deserved. He had devoted much of his life to their well-being by listening and talking to them all. But, as I said at the outset, he said little in print about himself. Not so his colleague Wilfred Bion, who was much more forthcoming.

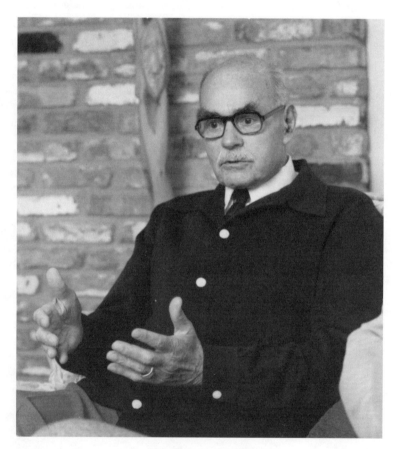

Wilfred Bion, 1976

6 Wilfred Bion: Group and Individual Analysis

Wilfred Bion was a giant. He was physically large and his influence remains immense. Particularly important are his insights about group and individual analysis, and about treating patients through attending to the feelings evoked in the analyst by their putting their inner images of themselves into him. Bion's resulting theories are often difficult to understand. But his account of their origin can be easily understood, beginning with his account of the feelings evoked by others' expectations of him as a boy and young man.

Early expectations[1]

Born on 8 September 1897 in Muttra in the United Provinces of north-west India (now Muthara, Uttar Pradesh), Wilfred Ruprecht Bion was the eldest of two children. His sister, Edna, was born three years later, in March 1901. She annoyed him by getting him into trouble with their parents. He also found his mother, Rhoda, difficult – warm one minute, suddenly cold the next. Most of all, however, he wrote of a bothersome inner 'Arf, Arfer' image of his father, Frederic, a civil service engineer. It was an amalgam, he wrote, of the braying, upper-class 'arf, arf, arf' laughter of members of his father's club; of the 'Our Father' prayer of his mother's Christian missionary family; and of his father's angry outbursts against him for his insatiable curiosity, like that of Rudyard Kipling's elephant's child.[2] He also remembered being terrified of not meeting others' expectations that he would become a famous big shot like his father who hunted with Edward James Corbett (mentioned in the *DNB*

as a 'destroyer of man-eating tigers'), King George V and General
Ironside. He remembered himself as a boy as being a 'sniveller
frightened even by the sight of a tiger trap'.[3] And he was frightened
too of England and of the expectation that he would become a hero
like those of the Indian Mutiny – Sir Henry Havelock and Sir James
Outram.

Nevertheless it was to England he was sent when he was eight,
when his mother took him to board at the prep school of Bishop's
Stortford College. She left him there, returned to India, and he did
not see her again for three years. On his first night he sobbed under
the bedclothes. One of the boys asked if he was homesick. But he
immediately realized from the boy's reaction that he must deny it. If
he must weep he must do so silently – like his mother, he wrote,
neither laughing nor crying. Years later he wrote of his misery at that
time to his son Julian, when he too went to prep school. He described
it as a 'sort of horrible sense of impending disaster . . . the 2 a.m.
feeling when some horrible worry comes on you with such force that
it makes your blood run cold'.[4]

Horrible worries included the prep school bully and the headmaster, particularly when the latter denounced one of the boys at
assembly for 'poisoning the mind of another'.[5] When the boy was
expelled Wilfred was convinced it was 'arf arfer' punishment for the
'wages of sin' of masturbating – 'wiggling'. He too was a masturba-
tor. What else could he do? It so comforted him, he wrote, 'as anything that brought relief in that dreadful darkness would have done'.[6]
Another comfort was friends – including two boys, Heaton Rhodes
and Dudley Hamilton, with whom he stayed in the holidays. But
again sex obtruded when, one evening, horseplaying with Wilfred on
going to bed, Dudley sensed Wilfred's sexual longing for him. From
then on Wilfred avoided Dudley at school. He could not bear his
tantalizing closeness.

Religion was no consolation. He hated the Church in the name of
which the school sanctioned its repression of sex. Rather than the
God of the Church, he deified the senior school's sports heroes. He
too became a hero – captain both of the school's water polo team
and of its rugger team. He was outstanding in every game except
cricket. But the glory of being school captain came too late. It was
eclipsed by the outbreak of war on 14 August 1914. Being a sports
hero hardly equalled being a war hero. And it was no compensation
for his failure in his late teens to win a scholarship to Oxford. Feeling
pressured by the wife of the prep school headmaster, with whom he
boarded that summer, and inspired by the sight of soldiers march-
ing past his school on his return there that autumn, he left the next
summer determined to join up.

But at the recruiting station in Lincoln's Inn, central London, he suffered the indignity of the recruiting officer dismissing him as a mere boy: 'You there – you with that college cap – 'op it'.[7] His father was 'flabbergasted' and used his influence to get him into officer training. Bion was sworn in on 4 January 1916, and no longer had to suffer the humiliation of being sneered at by a girl in the street who, only a few days before, had marked him out as a coward by giving him a white feather. Now, at last, he felt his mother was proud of him. He applied and was accepted in the Machine Gun Corps, and was commissioned as an officer to the 5th Tank Battalion. The unit left Southampton on 25 June 1917 for France, where his battalion was stationed near Ypres.

After getting hopelessly lost and immobilized in mud at the front on 25 September 1917, the batallion was almost totally obliterated in action near Metz on 20 November 1917. Bion's tank exploded. The crew found themselves in the enemy trenches they had been ordered to take. Bion continued to shoot at the enemy with a machine gun and, despite the rout, was recommended for the Victoria Cross (VC). The army, he wrote, was determined to find war heroes. And he was happy to be one, to spend the rest of his life 'basking in the warmth of approval'.[8]

But he also dreaded having to live up to others' expectations of him on being awarded the Distinguished Service Order (not the VC which, in the event, went posthumously to a man killed in the action of 20 November 1917). He had nightmares of not being the hero he was expected to be, and suffered the ignominy of feeling useless and frustrated in the Anglo-French offensive near Amiens on 8 August 1918. Angry with himself for not anticipating the dense mist rising from the river which engulfed the tank section during the advance into this action, he took out his irritation on a junior soldier, Sweeting, who had just had his chest blown to pieces. Years later Bion still remembered their ensuing conversation:

> 'Sir! Sir, why can't I cough?'
> What a question! What a time . . . I looked at his chest. His tunic was torn. No, it was not his tunic; the left side of his chest was missing . . .
> 'Mother . . . Mother . . . Mother . . .'. Then he saw me looking. 'Why can't I cough sir?'
> I could not stand it . . .
> 'Sweeting, *please* Sweeting . . . please, please *shut up*' . . .
> 'You will write to my mother? You *will* write sir, won't you?'[9]

'And then I think he died', Bion added. 'Or perhaps it was only me'. It killed his spirit. The horror haunted him on his return from France to London. Here, before joining his mother in Cheltenham, where his sister was at school, he went to Jermyn Street and, on having a Turkish bath, he fell asleep and again heard himself and Sweeting: 'Mother, Mother . . . You will write to my mother sir, won't you?'. 'No, blast you, I shan't! Shut up! Can't you see I don't want to be disturbed?'[10]

Bion also suffered nightmares about his nineteen-year-old second-in-command, Asser, also killed on 8 August, in his case for courageously refusing to surrender when the enemy surrounded his tank. Bion could not get over the fact that it was not Asser but himself who became a hero, including being decorated for his action that day with the French Legion of Honour, and with being mentioned in dispatches. They were a sham, Bion wrote, mere 'Hero dress'.[11] He never recovered. Most of what he most disliked about himself, he wrote, started then.[12]

It was his unjustified reputation as a hero, Bion modestly wrote, that led to his now being awarded the scholarship to read history which he had previously failed to win at Queen's College, Oxford. He started there at the beginning of 1919. But again he suffered the anxiety of not living up to others' expectations. He graduated in 1921, feeling a failure: he had not got the first-class degree his tutors expected of him; furthermore, he had won only a swimming Blue, not a rugger Blue as well (because he had a torn cartilage on the day of the Oxford–Cambridge match). Nevertheless he went on to play rugger for the famous Harlequins,[13] and was considered for an international cap.[14] On leaving Oxford, he went for a year to Poitiers University, but again he felt a failure, and that he had 'utterly wasted' his time there.[15]

From France he returned to England and to teaching at his old school, Bishop's Stortford College, where according to one of his pupils:

> [his arrival as] Master in the Christmas Term of 1922 caused a considerable sensation. Here came a young OS, just turned 25, built like an ox, with a distinguished athletic background and a fine war record: what would he be like as a Master? At first, frankly, he frightened us to death with his impassive face and brusque speech – and maybe in truth he was just as frightened of us. But fear didn't last long: it drained away, to be replaced by the greatest respect and in the end, for many of us, by adulation this side of idolatory.[16]

Another Old Stortfordian recalls reading parties from the school in Happisburgh, Norfolk, when Bion joined others in a gruelling tradition of New Year's swimming in the North Sea.

But Bion still felt a failure. The mother of one of his pupils accused him of sexually propositioning her son and Bion was dismissed. Bion blamed himself for not standing his ground and hiring a solicitor to contest the woman's charge. He also hated himself for what happened soon afterwards: he became engaged to the sister of a friend he was staying with, but she promptly jilted him for another man. Evidently, he concluded, he had not lived up to her expectations of him as a war hero.

Feeling utterly defeated he went into therapy. But that too was a failure. Bion expected the therapist to tackle his current problems, but instead he focused on the past. And, when he tried to help Bion become a therapist by referring him a patient, the patient failed to turn up. Bion nevertheless decided to pursue the idea of becoming a therapist and applied for medical training to UCL where, he wrote, he was accepted on the strength of his sports success. But again he quickly disappointed others' expectations of him by nearly failing his initial qualifying exams. Despite this, however, he went on to win a Gold Medal for surgery and graduated with honours.

On first qualifying in 1930, Bion worked for the Royal Air Force,[17] for what became the Maida Vale Hospital for Nervous Diseases, and for the Institute for the Scientific Treatment of Delinquency (formed in 1931 and now called the Portman Clinic). In the early 1930s he also joined the Tavistock Clinic, then located in Malet Place in Bloomsbury, and was rapidly promoted to be a senior staff member. His first patients there included the writer Samuel Beckett, referred because of various anxiety symptoms exacerbated by his father's death in July 1933.

A fellow Dubliner and doctor friend, Geoffrey Thompson, had suggested to Beckett that he have psychoanalysis, but it was illegal in Ireland. So Beckett came to London, where his treatment with Bion started in early 1934. It continued three times a week for nearly two years; Beckett accompanied Bion to Jung's lectures at the Tavistock in autumn 1935. Years later Bion said of his treatment of Beckett: 'I don't know that I did him much good. But I don't think I did him much harm either'.[18] Others said Beckett modelled his play, *Waiting for Godot*, on his therapy with Bion.

Whether or not Bion was Godot, he, like Beckett, was in therapy in the 1930s, first with one of his UCL teachers, Hadfield. Then, in 1937, he went into analysis with John Rickman (who, since 1934, had been in analysis with Klein). He also began training to become an analyst himself. Soon after his mother's death on 13 January 1939 he met an actress, Betty Jardine, on a three-week holiday in Happisburgh, and married her in April 1940. By then his analytic training and analysis with Rickman had stopped and the two men now found themselves working together as army officers running groups and writing about them.

Experiencing groups

Groups were the subject of Bion's very first published essay. It was included in a Tavistock collection of 1940, *The Neuroses of War*.[19] In it he noted ways in which one side in war seeks to distract the attention of the other from external danger by activating their inner phantasies, anxiety and guilt. Soldiers are more able than civilians to withstand this 'war of nerves', Bion wrote, because their training teaches them to subordinate concern for their individual safety to concern for the group. He accordingly argued that to counter the self-preoccupation of civilians with their inner fears and phantasies, they too should be organized like soldiers into groups so they could deal more effectively with the outer dangers of war.

In 1940 Bion joined the army High Command and was posted first to the Davy Hulme Military Hospital in Chester, and then to York. By early 1942 he was working as a senior psychiatrist with John Sutherland at a unit of the War Office Selection Board (WOSB) concerned with improving officer recruitment. Bion suggested organizing applicants into groups of eight or nine, and setting them a real task like building a bridge (the task Bion himself had when preparing for the offensive of 8 August 1918). From their performance on this task, he argued, applicants could be assessed in terms of their capacity to co-ordinate their individual interests in being selected with the interests of the group.[20]

The army liked the scheme in that it involved fellow soldiers (as well as psychiatrists) in officer selection; towards the end of summer 1942, the scheme's headquarters were moved closer to the War Office in London, to a country house called Wall Hall (nicknamed 'Valhalla'), near Watford. But Bion was not promoted to head the unit. As this meant he would not be able to decide which officers were selected, or to oversee training of incoming staff in his group selection methods, he asked for a transfer. This took him first to WOSB7 in Winchester (from March to August 1943) and in late 1943 to a wing run by Rickman in Hollymoor Hospital in Northfield, Birmingham, for rehabilitating soldiers suffering from neurosis. Here Rickman and Bion decided to develop a project Rickman had introduced in the Wharncliffe Emergency Hospital, Sheffield, and outlined in a memorandum written by Bion in 1940.[21]

On his arrival at Northfield, Bion found his work far from therapeutic. It was interrupted by patients and staff making one demand after another. Or they were apathetic. Either way, said Bion, every-one on the wing fled the task of tackling neurosis. To improve the situation he organized the men to deal with it as a shared group problem: just as in the army, for which the patients were being reha-bilitated, men are organized to meet the shared group problem of the enemy by leaders who are not afraid of what their men think of them, good or ill. Bion and Rickman accordingly organized the patients into activity groups, and into a large group scheduled to meet for half an hour every lunch-time, ostensibly for announcements but actually to think together about what was going on.

But very little, it seemed, went on. When Bion put this to the men they looked 'got at' by him. Soon afterwards they complained that the wards were dirty. This led to their organizing groups to clean them. Then a few complained that while they worked the rest were 'just a lot of shirkers',[22] 'skrim-shankers', 'work-shys' and malinger-ers. They ought to be punished.[23] Bion returned the problem to the men. He suggested they find a solution. But they were sceptical and ridiculed his suggestion by proposing they organize a dancing class. Taking in their challenge, and refusing to be daunted by it, Bion con-tinued to urge them to come up with concrete plans. Eventually they did. And, within a month, morale on the wing markedly improved. Bion's superiors, however, were not impressed. His hopes that, despite their likely opposition, they might eventually approve were soon dashed. Within six weeks of the experiment beginning, it was stopped. Bion left Birmingham and the next year he was posted to France.

Following the North Africa campaign and the finding that battle-scarred men got worse on being sent home, it was decided they should be treated closer to the front. It was for this purpose that Bion was sent to France in June 1944, after the allied landings in Normandy, as the psychiatrist most likely to be acceptable to Field Marshal Montgomery. It was in Normandy that he learnt from his wife of the birth, on 27 February 1945, of their daughter Parthenope, called after the old name for Naples used by Virgil in *The Georgics*. But within hours of writing to Bion of Parthenope's birth, Betty was dead. Perhaps her death was due to septicaemia or to a pulmonary embolism, neither of which could be effectively treated in the Bournemouth nursing home where Parthenope was born.

Bion was devastated. He returned to England and spent the rest of the year working for WOSB in Sanderstead, Surrey. WOSB's work now involved not so much officer selection as reclassifying, rede-ploying and resettling men as civilians when the war ended. For Bion, return to civilian life included giving up the flat in Pond Street, Hampstead, which he had shared with Betty. He now moved to Iver

Heath, near Slough, Berkshire, with his widowed father (who lived until February 1949), Parthenope and with the Ransoms, a family who had looked after her during the war.

From Iver Heath he commuted to London, where his work now included seeing private patients in his consulting-room at 99 Harley Street. He also resumed his psychoanalytic training and again went into analysis, not least because he was worried about his reaction to Parthenope. Still grieving over his wife's death, he could hardly bear to take in their daughter's demands. His resistance culminated one weekend when, sitting in the garden, he could see that Parthenope wanted him. She called out to him, crawled towards him and became increasingly distressed. But he refused to budge and forbade the nurse to pick her up. Appalled, the nurse overrode his order and took Parthenope into her arms. Then the spell broke. But, Bion added, 'I had lost the child. . . . It was a shock, a searing shock, to find such depth of cruelty in myself'. It made him think of Hamlet telling Ophelia, 'Nymph, in thy orisons be all my sins remembered'.[24] Perhaps he looked to find an analyst to be his Ophelia. His having worked so closely with Rickman as a fellow officer in the war precluded his going back into analysis with him. Instead he applied to Klein, who took him on and whom he appreciated for not being deflected by his outward 'masculine excellence' from seeing what was going on inside.

At the end of the war he also returned to the Tavistock which, following its wartime evacuation to Hampstead, was now housed in 2 Beaumont Street, west London. Here, on 5 October 1945, he was unanimously elected chair of its planning committee. He also became involved in running therapy groups as part of the Tavistock's involvement in pioneering out-patient psychiatric treatment in the new National Health Service. The groups he ran consisted of eight patients meeting for two one-and-a-half-hour sessions each week. They felt immensely secure, wrote Eric Trist, a clinical psychologist Bion invited to join him in running a group, because Bion was so 'large . . . warm, utterly imperturbable and inexhaustibly patient'. Trist himself, however, found the work depressing because the patients were so disturbed. He wanted to give up. But Bion dissuaded him, saying that that was what the patients wanted. The answer was not to give up but to take in and work with what the patients made him feel.[25]

Adopting this approach himself, Bion noted that group members made him feel the centre of their attention. They looked to him to be a leader – a god. No one else would do. But they were also disappointed in him. Bion called this constellation of expectations and disappointments an inwardly shared 'basic assumption'. It was a phantasy that contradicted the group's outward avowed aim of working together to solve their shared problems. In this state of mind, Bion noted, on the basis of the feelings it evoked in him, the group wants magic and religion. It is hostile to learning from experience. It does not want science or knowledge. It dismisses the leader's attempts at understanding as cold and heartless abstraction. Or the group splits into two – one subgroup agrees on depending on the leader, and the other is so exacting in its pursuit of knowledge that it fails to recruit others to its cause. Or – and again Bion drew on the feelings groups produced in him – group members retreat from outward work into an inward phantasy of meeting together to fight or take flight from a common enemy. Alternatively, they retreat into an inward phantasy: two members of the group pair off to give birth to a messiah who will solve all the group's problems.

Bion described these 'dependent', 'fight–flight' and 'pairing' 'basic assumption' phantasies in his first book, *Experiences in Groups*. It was published in 1961. In it he also described the group analyst's experience of being made the outward repository of the group members' shared inner ideas:

> The analyst feels he is being manipulated so as to be playing a part, no matter how difficult to recognize, in somebody else's phantasy – or he would do if it were not for what in recollection I can only call a temporary loss of insight, a sense of experiencing strong feelings and at the same time a belief that their existence is quite adequately justified by the objective situation.[26]

Group members, Bion argued, resort to phantasies and they try to get the group leader, as an outside figure, to take on these phantasies rather than investigate, discover and face what is actually going on, which, they feel, might lead to disaster. They dread discovering something as catastrophic as Oedipus discovered on questioning the Sphinx – that he had murdered his father and married his mother. Panic at what they might discover prevents group members from thinking and talking coherently. Instead they become determined to build a Tower of Babel. They fragment into schisms in seeking to achieve phantasies of being safe in dependency and messianic hopes of reaching heaven.

Group and organizational management consultancy and therapy have been enormously influenced by Bion's work, but he himself had little faith in groups as a means of therapy or cure. All they had ever cured him of, he quipped, was the expectation that they might take kindly to his efforts. He was much more hopeful of individual analysis, to which he now increasingly devoted himself. In 1948, as well as chairing the Medical Section of the British Psychological Society, he was accepted as an Associate Member of the British Psycho-Analytical Society, and on 1 November 1950 presented a paper for full membership of the society about his analysis of a man bordering on madness. A few months later, aged fifty-three, he also fell in love.

Love and madness

Bion first caught sight of Francesca McCallum, the woman who became his second wife, in the Tavistock refectory in mid-March 1951. She was twenty-eight. After training in singing since 1940 and studying economics and statistics at Exeter University, she had worked at the War Office in London and then at GCHQ in Cairo. Here, in early March 1945, she had married and, on returning to England after the war, continued studying music and began professional engagements singing opera, oratorio and lieder. In April 1949 she was suddenly widowed: the plane of which her husband was test pilot exploded in mid-air. She fulfilled her singing engagements for the rest of the year. But she had lost heart and, through a friend in the War Office, got a job working for Elliott Jaques on a project on worker–management relations which he was doing for Glacier Metals at the Tavistock.

'Being terribly formal', Francesca says, Bion asked a mutual colleague, Ken Rice, to introduce them. Through the next few weeks they met a great deal. Bion also wrote her love letters almost every day, including the day they married, 9 June 1951. Having settled in Redcourt, East Croydon, with six-year-old Parthenope, they had two more children: Julian, born on 30 July 1952; and Nicola, born on 13 June 1955.

A colleague of Bion's once told Francesca she was 'nurturing genius' in marrying Bion.[27] As for Bion, he was nurturing, or at least analysing, patients suffering from varying degrees of madness. During the 1950s he wrote of working with patients whom psychosis stripped of all love, life and feeling, and who, as a result, often seemed psychologically dead. He had described just such a patient in his paper of 1950. Called 'The imaginary twin', it was about a teacher, tall like him, who had long fended off life and anxiety with a number of dreary, rule-bound obsessive rituals. These included having to rest his head on his hand at night to stop it touching the pillow, not shaking hands and compulsively washing them to get rid of contaminating contact with others. Since years of therapy had failed to help, he had been recommended brain surgery. To avoid this option he decided to try psychoanalysis and was referred to Bion.

For months his analysis threatened to be as ineffective as his previous therapy. He responded desultorily to Bion interpreting Oedipal conflicts in him. He did not begin to come alive until Bion took note of the feelings stirred up within him by the patient. These included, he wrote, 'an overpowering sense of boredom and depression', alternating with an almost jocular effect when the patient paused as if to say, 'Go on; it's your turn'.[28] Bion also noted the patient's anxiety whenever this rhythm was broken, and his sense of futility when the rhythm continued with the psychoanalytic interpretations he also invited and expected.

When Bion put this to the patient, he responded the next day by saying he wondered whether it was worth continuing. Perhaps, Bion replied, analysis was not the solution; perhaps he needed a different analyst; or perhaps he saw Bion only to have someone to go to. At this the patient told an anecdote about a woman he knew who always complained of one thing or another. Recently she had complained of rheumatic pain. He had fobbed her off by suggesting she take Amytal. Other times he told anecdotes beginning 'I was thinking of talking to Mr X and telling him . . .'; what followed would be an account of a man like himself. It was the same with Bion. He treated Bion's comments either as vague complaints to be fobbed off with sleep-inducing Amytal indifference, or he warded off his resentment of Bion by treating him as a Mr X twin of himself, jocularly evading what he said.

When Bion put this to him, the patient replied that he felt tired and unclean. Bion explained that this was because he had now taken back into himself his jocular and complaining self which he had previously put into Bion. It was bringing together these two aspects within himself that made him feel tired and unclean. But it also helped bring together other aspects of himself. He now dreamt he parked his car too close to a menacing Bion-like figure. It made him feel blocked and trapped. But in dreaming and telling his dream, he faced these previously externalized aspects of himself coming together within him. They thereby became more integrated – a process which he had previously warded off with his contact-avoiding rituals.

Generalizing from the feelings evoked in him by this man and by other patients, Bion argued that it is dread of depression resulting from bringing together aspects of the self that leads in madness, or schizophrenia, to their being externalized into others. Another example was a patient who, dreading knowing and thinking what he felt, experienced Bion as doing the knowing and thinking. But then he felt Bion had stolen his thinking, and would hate and attack him were he to take it back.[29]

Rather than think or know or experience what is going on inside, wrote Bion, the schizophrenic pushes these aspects of himself into others outside. An instance was a patient who, through the first twenty minutes of a session, made Bion feel increasingly frightened, especially because of what he already knew about this patient. He feared that the patient was thinking of attacking him. Putting this into words, he said, 'You have been pushing into my insides your fear that you will murder me'. The patient remained silent, clenching his fists until his knuckles went white. But as he did so the tension between them subsided. Bion commented, 'When I spoke to you, you took your fear that you would murder me back into yourself; you are now feeling afraid you will make a murderous attack on me'.[30] That was why he clenched his fist – to stop himself giving vent to the thought and feeling he now acknowledged as his, namely his impulse to attack Bion.

Writing further about the thoughts and feelings such patients evoke, Bion noted that, in attacking and fragmenting their feeling and thinking, schizophrenics often externalize the resulting fragments, turning them into outwardly attacking and retaliating 'bizarre objects'. As bits-and-pieces thing-like fragments they cannot be integrated or brought together. They can only be amassed, 'agglomerated' or 'compressed'.[31]

Fragmenting thinking, Bion noted, can also involve attacking links between thoughts. An example was a patient who, after arriving fifteen minutes late for a session, paused for a long time, turning restlessly from side to side. Bion's account of the patient is as follows:

I don't suppose I shall do anything today. I ought to have rung my mother. Another pause. Then

No; I thought it would be like this.

Again he paused, this time for some time, before saying

Nothing but filthy things and smells . . . I think I've lost my sight.[32]

Bion put the fragments together with the feelings the man had previously evoked in him. The patient's attacking with pauses the links between one thought and the next and his resulting inability to think, which the patient called losing his sight, were attempts to rid himself of something painful. That was why he turned restlessly from side to side. He was frightened that if he took thinking and seeing back into himself he would be overwhelmed. That was why he replied to Bion

with the words 'My head is splitting; maybe my dark glasses', referring to the dark glasses Bion had worn in a previous session. That
was why he said 'I ought to have rung my mother' at the beginning
of the session, referring not only to his resistance to getting together
with his mother or with anyone else, but also to his resistance to
bringing his thoughts together within him for fear of the damage that
might result.

But what happens when attacking links between thoughts and
getting rid of them into others fails? A case in point, wrote Bion, was
a patient who prevented this from happening by leaving out pro-
nouns, verbs and other connecting words from what he said. It
prevented any understanding or 'coupling', as Bion put it, between
them. Bion began to understand what was going on when one day
the patient wondered out loud how Bion could stand it. Evidently,
Bion concluded, talking for this man was less a matter of connecting words grammatically than putting feelings he could not stand into
Bion, so Bion could stand them. He hoped, Bion speculated, that
they could thereby be changed through 'sojourning' in Bion's mind.
But this also failed because the patient prevented it by arrogantly
deriding as stupid any attempt to thus communicate through feelings rather than words.[33]

Others retreat into seeing things that are not there. An example
was a patient recovering from schizophrenia who became convinced
that Bion wanted to murder him. The next session he began by
quickly glancing at Bion before mechanically matching his pace to
Bion's as they each walked to their place in the consulting-room.
The patient then sat down on the couch and stared fixedly into the
corner of the room. There it seemed he saw the murderous version
of himself that he had put into Bion the previous day and which he
had just taken back into himself with his opening glance. Staring into
the corner he ejected and deposited it there – a process of visually
taking things in and ejecting them which he represented in a dream
he told Bion the next day of swallowing him and then losing him as
he slept.[34]

Bion saw this patient and others in his London consulting-room,
which he rented at 135 Harley Street from 1958 to 1963. Travelling
there from Redcourt on 2 February 1959 he fainted at Victoria
station. He was hospitalized in St George's for tests. While there
he worked on an essay, 'Attacks on linking', which became one of
his most important and enduringly influential. In dwelling on the
mothering precursors of Klein's 'projective identification' process,
whereby patients put their feeling and thinking into the analyst, it
marked a new departure in Kleinian theory and practice.

Mothering inside out

Perhaps Bion was mindful of Francesca mothering the children –
now aged fourteen, six and three – when, in 'Attacks on linking', he
compared the analyst's experience of taking in his patient's feelings
with that of the mother taking in her children's feelings. He illustrated the point by describing a patient affectionately remembering
how his mother used to cope with him as a difficult child. As the
patient told Bion about this memory, he stammered. Another time
the patient spoke of a girl whom he had met and who seemed to
understand him but then he moved convulsively as if to stab and kill
the idea of her understanding him. At other times, fearful of dying,
the patient sought to get rid of this fear into Bion. But he felt that
Bion resisted taking in his fear, just as he felt his mother had resisted
taking in his fears as a child. Or his fears completely overwhelmed
her. His stammering and convulsive movements, however, also indicated a contrary tendency: he so envied his mother or anyone else
taking in and understanding him that he attacked and destroyed the
very idea.[35]

When this happens, Bion wrote, the patient does not credit others
with thinking and understanding but imagines them as only taking in
his thoughts and feelings so as to greedily devour and destroy them.
Others thereby become greedily devouring figures in the patient's
mind. Bion claimed that this makes the patient sever and attack ever
more harshly his links with them. An example was a patient who,
severing all links, made others and his feelings into disconnected
inanimate objects with his fragmented utterance: 'Rain – without a
raincoat – taking the only taxi – pneumonia feared for me – self in rain
at my house. . . . baby with a horn on its nose – some cowl on its head
– his wife and blood – shambles'.[36] Bion could take in his words, but
the patient's attack on what was alive and going on psychologically
between them made it difficult to digest or understand.

Bion spoke further of analytic understanding and not understanding, and its parallels with early mothering, in a talk to the psychoanalytic congress in Edinburgh in 1961. Suppose, he said, the
baby expects the mother – or her breast – but finds her gone. If
the baby can bear frustration, his expectation – or 'pre-conception'
– becomes a thought. It helps to bridge the gap between wanting and
satisfaction. Freud wrote similarly of the hungry baby, faced with the
mother's absence, hallucinating her presence. This is the origin,
Freud claimed, of the hallucinations of dreams. To this Bion added
that if the baby cannot bear frustration his preconception becomes
not a thought but a thing. It becomes a bad object, a 'bad breast', fit

only to be ejected with the result that learning from experience is evaded; or it is replaced with substituted omniscience.

Ordinarily, Bion went on, babies act so as to arouse in the mother feelings they want to eject. By accepting these feelings the mother enables the baby to take them back as acceptable and bearable by her. But if she cannot accept the feelings the baby seeks to arouse in her, he escalates his efforts to eject them but in doing so he develops an image of her as greedily stripping the meaning away from everything he puts into her. It leaves him feeling empty and starved of understanding. In analysis it takes the form of the patient feeling that the analyst strips everything he puts into him of its meaning, so that he is quite unable to experience the analyst as understanding, helpful or good.

In mothers, said Bion, understanding includes the capacity for 'reverie', for taking in the baby's sensations of himself and converting them into what can be experienced psychologically. Using a term he had mentioned in a letter to Francesca in March 1960, when she was looking after the children in a cottage they had bought that year in Trimingham in Norfolk, Bion called this process of conversion 'alpha-function'; other times he called the resulting alpha-elements 'idées mères'.[37] Without them, he wrote, we can neither think nor dream. This can happen if the mother is unable to take in the baby's self-sensations. They are then liable to remain or become stripped of psychological content, thereby constituting what Bion called unknown and unknowable 'beta-elements'. If the mother is unable to take in and bear her baby's fearful self-sensations – in extremis his sense of himself as dying – then the baby has no option but to take them back into himself, stripped of meaning not as fear made bearable, wrote Bion, but as 'nameless dread'.

In his book Learning from Experience, published in 1962, Bion wrote more about the parallels between the mother taking in, or 'containing' as he now put it, her baby's self-sensations and the analyst containing the patients' self-sensations. He likened the process to taking in, metabolizing and digesting food. He also likened it to a woman taking in her lover's penis in sex. Bion now developed a notation for recording this outside-in process. He used the letters 'L', 'H' and 'K' to stand schematically for the links of love, hate and knowledge between mother and child, analyst and patient. He likened his schematization of these links to what the mathematician and philosopher Jules Henri Poincaré called 'selected facts'. In Elements of Psychoanalysis (1963) Bion developed his notation into a mathematical co-ordinate system or 'Grid'.

Bion was also interested in painting, calling those he did in his and Francesca's first home in East Croydon 'mere daubs'. He continued painting and drawing after their move, in 1963, to Wells Rise, near Primrose Hill, where he now, for the first time, saw patients in a consulting-room in his own house. From 1956 to 1962 he had been Director of the London Clinic of Psycho-Analysis; in 1962 he became President of the British Psycho-Analytical Society, a position he held until 1966. In letters to his children he described this involving him being treated as a 'Big Noise' – a 'sort of psychoanalytic Pope', as he also put it at the society's jubilee celebrations of 1963. His experience of presiding over the Society's Connaught Rooms dinner celebrating the publication in English of Freud's collected works in 1966 is delightfully depicted in a letter to his then eleven-year-old daughter Nicola, in which he drew the faces of the assembled company as 'plaice on a fish-monger's slab'.[38]

Drawing and painting also feature in Bion's books. He began his book *Transformations*, published in 1965, for instance, with a reflection on Monet's transformation of his experience of a poppy field into an Impressionist painting. He compared it to the analyst transforming into words his experience of what goes on between himself and the patient. He argued that it involves the analyst seeking the origin – 'O' – of the patient's behaviour and its transformation. In schizophrenics this may involve the patient talking as if there was no way 'O' could be transformed. The book also dwells on the recent shift of focus in psychoanalysis: from treating the barrier between the conscious and unconscious mind in the neurotic to treating the effects on the schizophrenic of variously putting his image of himself into the analyst and barring himself from putting it there. He likened this shift to that which had taken place in modern physics in terms of Werner Heisenberg's uncertainty principle. He also described picturing what goes on between patient and analyst in terms of myths, stories and plays, using as examples Oedipus at the crossroads, the Mad Hatter's tea party from Lewis Carroll and Pirandello's *Six Characters in Search of an Author* (a London production of which he saw in 1964). He ended *Transformations* by likening the analyst's task to Bishop Berkeley's account of Newton dealing with 'ghosts of departed qualities' in differential calculus. He also likened analysis to what St John of the Cross and other mystics had achieved in transforming 'O' – our essence or ultimate being – into words.

On 11 October 1967 Bion gave a talk to fellow members of the Melanie Klein Trust (of which he was President from 1966 to 1967), stating that, to be maximally responsive to the non-sensuous psychological reality of what happens between himself and the patient, the analyst must empty himself of all sense impressions of memories of the past and wishes for the future.[39] He reiterated this injunction in his next book, *Attention and Interpretation*, published in 1970. In it he also noted the neurotic's inner resistance to analysis and the schizophrenic's externalizing evocation of the analyst's resistance; through evoking in the analyst his memory, desire and quest for understanding, the schizophrenic obstructs the analyst's experience of what is going on between them. To characterize the analyst's success in nevertheless freeing himself from memory and desire, Bion used Keats's expression 'negative capability' – an expression Keats had used to designate bearing with 'uncertainties, mysteries, doubts, without any irritable reaching after fact and reason', an attribute he found pre-eminently in Shakespeare.[40] Free from memory, desire and understanding, Bion concluded, still using the analogy of mothering, psychoanalysis constitutes 'the restoration of god (the Mother) and the evolution of god (the formless, infinite, ineffable, non-existent)'.[41]

American exodus

In April 1967 Bion gave lectures in Los Angeles. One of them illustrated the process by which inner images are externalized into the analyst with a fifty-three-year-old patient who began with a torrent of know-all free associations and then expected Bion to be the know-all, to instantly understand everything about him.[42] Back in London, Bion felt 'hedged in'[43] – 'throttled', according to Marion Milner[44] – by the Kleinians there. He wanted to get away. That autumn Francesca looked for a house for them in California and on 25 January 1968 they arrived in Los Angeles and settled in Brentwood, inland from Santa Monica. Their children stayed at school in England, Julian (then fifteen) at Harrow and Nicola (then twelve) at Westonbirt. Parthenope had already left England in 1963 for Italy. Here, after studying in Florence, she took a degree in philosophy in Rome and married Luigi Talamo, a viola player in the Rome opera orchestra. She trained as an analyst and eventually settled with Luigi in Turin.

In the early 1970s Bion and Francesca bought a holiday home in the Dordogne, but they continued to live mostly in Los Angeles, where Bion continued painting and seeing patients – at first ten, then eight, a day. They included several analysts who wanted a training analysis with him.[45] He also gave seminars and lectures at conferences, later admitting that he was often discomfited by his audiences expecting him to be a 'sort of messiah or deity',[46] with their 'Bion–Bion–Bion' accolades.[47] In his lectures and seminars he talked, as he had long written, about treating patients through attending to the feelings they evoked in him. In the 1960s he had written about this in often difficult, pared-down abstractions. In his talks in the

1970s, however, he illustrated the processes involved much more fully, with easily understandable everyday examples.

In lectures in São Paulo in 1973, for instance, he illustrated the parallel between analysts and mothers containing or not containing feelings put into them by others in terms of the mother who, disturbed by her baby's crying, exasperatedly reacts by saying, 'I don't know what's the matter with the child!' Faced with her exasperation, said Bion, the baby has no option but to take back his crying and disturbance undigested. Alternatively the mother may pick up the baby and comfort him so he feels that, by screaming and yelling, he has got rid of his feelings of impending disaster into her. By picking him up and comforting him the mother enables the baby to take back his feelings and find them much more bearable than the disaster with which his yelling began. Bion further illustrated the point with an anecdote told him by Sue Isaacs-Elmhirst (see p. 34 above), who was also living at this time in Los Angeles. She described a baby saying, 'oo el, oo el', which turned out to be his means of taking in and comforting himself with his mother's soothing 'well, well' words when she was gone.[48]

Bion also illustrated his theories with clinical examples. Made mindful perhaps of students in the early 1970s by his son Julian being a medical student and by his daughter Nicola studying French and Spanish at New Hall, Cambridge (1973–6), Bion lectured in Rio de Janeiro in 1974 about a twenty-one-year-old student he had treated in London. After several meetings Bion put it to the student that neither of them seemed to know why he came, to which the student replied, 'I thought you knew. My difficulty is that I blush terribly. I thought you would have noticed it by this time'.[49] Outwardly, though, his face was completely wan. There was no blushing to be seen. It was inside. Or it was inside Bion. The student felt sure Bion knew about it. He felt sure everybody knew about it. That was why he stopped seeing his friends – because he could not bear them seeing and taking his blushing in.

In clinical seminars in Brasilia in 1975 Bion discussed other examples:[50] an eighteen-year-old's fear that his analyst might become a horrifying and dangerous ghost of his dead father, who had been a doctor; a woman fearful that her analyst's fame might prevent him from stooping to get close to what she felt inside; a diplomat so fearful of giving away important information which his analyst could use against him that he made what he said into rubbish; a patient who put into his analyst his envious wish to destroy his brother's ability as a doctor, with the result that he pictured his analyst enviously seeking to destroy and confuse him. In another seminar Bion talked of a patient's flood of information evoking in the analyst the drive to answer with a flood of interpretations.

Bion urged his colleagues to tolerate the 'emotional disturbance' evoked in them by their patients. At a conference in Topeka in March 1976 he warned against normalizing, deifying and assimilating those who disturb everyday reality with their insights by saying 'Yes, you are a god like us'.[51] Possibly thinking of his four-year-old grandchild Alessandra, born in 1972, he also talked at Topeka of the caesura of birth, and the psychological continuity between being in and outside the womb.

This theme recurred in Bion's weekly discussions in April 1976 at the Brentwood Veterans Administration Hospital in which – approvingly quoting Maurice Blanchot's dictum 'La réponse est le malheur de la question' – he warned against forestalling with premature answers what goes on between the patient and analyst in analysis. He recommended the skill of Wilfred Trotter, his University College Hospital surgery teacher during the 1920s, in listening to his patients – aristocrats and commoners alike – and he insisted, with Darwin, that 'it is fatal to reason whilst observing, though so necessary beforehand and so useful afterwards'.[52]

Bion illustrated the need to suspend reasoning – to attend, listen and wait – with a patient he had treated in the early 1960s,[53] whose problems began after he left school and started work as a research chemist. At his first session the patient could not speak for stammering. Its noise filled the silence. So did other noises: his deep breathing in and out, his swallowing, his straining to fart. His refusal to talk evoked Bion's arrogance. How dare this man keep him waiting for the words he wanted! The patient's 'spluttering and farting and sucking away with his lips', wrote Bion, evoked the image of a one-man-band. His various organs – mouth, anus, throat and lips – wanted to be heard all at once. The patient agreed: 'they were trying to settle who was top'.[54] Bion saying so freed him to talk without stammering – to talk of the various aspects of himself that wanted to put others down, including Bion and his colleagues at work.

Returning to São Paulo in April 1978, Bion again spoke about analysts treating patients through attending to the feelings they evoke in them. Examples included an eighteen-year-old anorexic, who countered her fear of being invaded and controlled by her father by evoking the feeling in others (including Bion) that she was 'very beautiful, like a distant star . . . very far away . . . whom nobody would dare to approach'.[55] He also talked of the puzzlement left in him by a patient whose mother and siblings had all been murdered one night when he was a baby; he went on to have terrifying nightmares and became terrified by his own cruelty, which included recently tripping up and badly injuring a girl in the street. What did it mean? Why did he do it? How was it connected with the murder? The puzzle remained.

Sometimes, Bion indicated in an essay published the next February, the puzzle remains because of the obstacles put in the way of the analyst taking in what is going on between him and the patient. The analyst's task, he wrote, is like that of the army officer faced with having to think under fire.[56] Perhaps he was remembering himself as an army officer in the First World War. Certainly, from the early 1970s, he was very much involved in writing up his First World War memoirs, not only in an autobiography but in three autobiographical novels.

The novels describe taking in and becoming the container of other people's expectations and feelings. *The Dream* (1975) concerns a couple faced with having to deal with an invading army; in *The Past Presented* (1977) a character is taken over by her maid. All three novels, and particularly *The Dawn of Oblivion* (1979), show how Bion was taken over and invaded by the boy he was in India, in prep and public school, and by himself as a man telling himself to be a hero, 'Stand up! Be erect! Oh great and fallacious Phallus!'[57] The novels also depict him being invaded by the ghosts of his First World War tank battalion, by himself as a doctor and analyst, and by his patients including the blushing student (see p. 130 above). He compared the effect to the grin left by the absent Cheshire Cat in *Alice's Adventures in Wonderland*.

At the end of July 1979 Bion and Francesca moved from Brentwood to a hotel in Los Angeles, where they bought a flat, planning to spend half of each year there and the other half in England. They wanted to be closer to their children: to Parthenope and her family in Italy (where, tragically, on 16 July 1998, she and her younger daughter Patrizia, then aged eighteen, were killed in a car accident); to Julian (who now works as an anaesthetist in Birmingham); and to Nicola (who worked for many years in publishing in Oxford). On 1 September they returned to London, where Bion saw patients and gave supervisions. He arranged to continue this work in Abingdon, near Oxford, on moving there on 5 October. But less than a month later, on 1 November, he was diagnosed as having myeloid leukaemia.

The same day Isabel Menzies Lyth (who has been particularly influential in applying Bion's Kleinian ideas in analysing groups and organizations) had arranged to begin supervision with him. Instead, she and her analyst husband, Oliver, visited him in hospital. Bion did not tell them the diagnosis. He simply remarked, 'Life is full of surprises, mostly unpleasant'. That afternoon he was reading M. M.

Kaye's blockbuster *The Far Pavilions*. It had been given him by his son, Julian, and is about a man faced, as Bion was, with others' expectations of him as an Indian-born Englishman. He was deeply moved by the story, as he had often been before in comparing the *Bhagavad Gita*, and its philosophical dialogue about war between Krishna and Arjuna, to what goes on between analyst and patient in analysis. He had hoped to go to India later that year – for the first time since leaving it when he was eight. But a week after his initial diagnosis with leukaemia he died, on 8 November 1979.

Five years before, he had written to Julian about the widespread aversion to attending to what goes on between doctors, patients and others: 'for some reason', he noted, 'when "mind meets mind", or "boy meets girl", or "boy meets boy" ', people 'shy off it as if shot'.[58] If doctors and therapists nowadays less often shy off the inside-out processes involved, this is largely thanks to Bion. It is also thanks to Esther Bick, whose contribution to psychoanalysis is the subject of the next chapter.

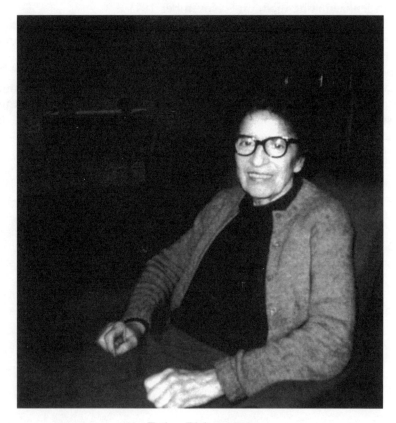

Esther Bick, *c.*1960

7 Esther Bick: Infant Observation

Esther Bick is notable for highlighting the importance of observing mothers and babies as means of becoming aware of the inner world driving our outer behaviour. Like many developments in psychoanalysis, Bick's insights come to us largely by word of mouth and from written accounts of her work by those she knew and supervised and most of all from those attending the seminars she ran for students to discuss their findings. These sources all testify to Bick's devotion to infant observation and her teaching of it being and continuing to be immensely inspiring.

Bick herself left little written record either of her work or of her life. From what little remains, it seems that her infancy was very happy but that this was followed by years of considerable hardship. Perhaps it was a quest to recover her early years that led her to initiate infant observation training. This initiative in turn led her to discover ways in which, for lack of feeling inwardly mothered as babies, children and adults may cling to an outer surface or skin.

Polish refugee[1]

Esther Bick, or 'Nusia' as she was known to her friends, was born Esteza Lifsza Wander on 4 July 1902 into an extremely poor, very religious Jewish family living in the country near Przemyśl in Galicia on the Ukrainian border of the Austro-Hungarian Empire. Her mother suffered a breakdown at the time of her birth, so Esther had to be wetnursed and brought up by her grandparents. She adored them, especially her grandmother whom she remembered into old age with enormous affection and love.

But her early happiness with her grandmother soon ended. When she was five her grandmother became pregnant and Esther was returned to her mother. Her mother too was pregnant – with Esther's brother. Many years later Esther recalled how, when she first learnt of his imminent arrival, she suddenly wet her pants (an experience she came to feel illustrated the precariousness of our inward sense of being held together being easily upset by sudden shock). His birth was followed five years later by the birth of a sister who died when Esther was still a child. She blamed her sister's death on her mother and was determined to get away. She studied Hebrew and planned on settling in Israel. More immediately, on finishing school when she was twelve, she was employed by a farmer. She worked for him on his land in the morning, and taught his children in the afternoon. She also persuaded a friend to attend a course with her in nursery school teaching, which had recently started in the nearby town. Later she criticized the course for being purely theoretical and not requiring any practical and direct experience of being with young children.

Having nevertheless passed the course's exams, Esther suffered further hardship. Her father had been sent to Siberia during the First World War, and had returned home very ill, soon after which he died. But nobody told Esther. When she found out she was furious. It made her more determined than ever to get away. As her mother's oldest child, however, she had to stay in the area to support the family, which she now did by working and teaching Hebrew in a home for girls orphaned by the war. She very much enjoyed the work, perhaps because it reminded her of her own infancy. 'I had a lovely room', she later recalled, 'and everything I needed'. She loved watching the little girls with their nursery school teacher. It decided her to study child psychology. She got a student to teach her chemistry and maths, and taught herself the other subjects – including history, Greek and Latin – needed to qualify her for university entrance. She wanted to study in Switzerland because of the work Piaget was doing on child psychology there, but there was no way she could do so in view of the restrictions on immigration and employment. The same obstacles prevented her from becoming a student in Germany and Austria. But a rich friend in Vienna persuaded her that she could find some means of supporting herself there, which she did, again by looking after children. 'And it was so cold, and I had no gloves', she later recalled. 'On top of that, the father of this child started to make advances to me, so I left them and went on'.[2]

The Latin Esther had taught herself won her a university place. But the fees, especially for foreigners, were very high. Again she had to find paid work, including working in a children's home run by Marianne Prager from 1930 to 1936. Some time during this period she met and married a medical student, Philip Bick. Around 1934 she became an assistant to the child psychologist Charlotte Bühler.

Bühler was then engaged, as one of her other students put it, in 'making detailed studies of development in babies on the basis of meticulous and minute obervations from birth onwards'.[3] She wanted to develop 'baby tests' – norms of behaviour against which to assess children up to the age of six. Unable to collect such data through the Vienna hospital system, she arranged for her assistants and students to record the behaviour of inmates in a home for unwanted and neglected infants. In her interview with Sandra Mancia, Bick remembered (speaking in English which she felt uncomfortable using because it marked her out as a foreigner) that as one of Bühler's assistants, she had to 'find six to eight months babies, put them in a playpen, one is A and the other one is B, there is a stopwatch. After a minute you see what A does to B and what B does to A, and make such an arrow, A to B and B to A'.[4] It was all outward stuff: 'really behaviouristic', she said, 'just terrible'. She had to use a stopwatch to study twins, and count their social responses to each other. It was this, she later maintained, that first led her to want to study 'the ordinary life' of babies in their own 'family environment'.[5]

But any prospect of implementing this plan after gaining her doctorate in 1936 was halted by the German invasion of Vienna on 12 March 1938. Esther's husband, Philip, from whom she was later divorced, and who was then in his last year studying medicine, helped her escape from the Gestapo into Switzerland. As a foreigner, she still could not get work there, and was sent by a Miss Hauser from the refugee camp to stay with her sister, Eva, in London.

Here Esther earned £2 a week doing housework. Inspired by a fellow refugee's account of his analysis in Vienna, she also sought analysis. Her fellow Vienna student, Ilse Hellman, who was now working in a child guidance clinic established by Bühler in London, recommended an Anna Freudian analyst. But Esther hated her for assuming that if she lost her job she would expect analysis for free. The analyst was 'rubbish', she later said, a 'bitch'. After a couple of months with this analyst Esther made her excuses and left. She then went to see her fellow refugee's analyst. But he too was no good. He would not take her on because, he said, she was too mentally ill.

Esther was rescued by a grandmotherly figure, just as she had been as a baby. Through the Society of British University Women, to which she now belonged, she took up the offer of a two-week holiday, in July 1939, on the country estate, near Sudbury, of a Miss Violet Oates. She was the sister of Captain Oates, famed for having walked out into the snow to die rather than delay his companions on the return journey of Scott's disastrous 1910–12 Antarctic expedition.

Violet was even more impressive than her brother, in Esther's opinion. She was so 'nice', 'wonderful, wonderful'. She too was a victim of a 'bitchy' mother, she said. Her mother had stopped her marrying the man she loved. Still a spinster, she was wonderfully friendly and welcoming, invited Esther's friend Eva Hauser to stay too, and kept them both on – Eva to work in the garden, and Esther to serve at table. She stayed there until Christmas 1939 and then went to join her Vienna friend and colleague Marianne Prager, who was working in a hostel for refugee boys in Manchester. Here Esther found a job as a maid looking after a child. She also again sought analysis – this time with Michael Balint, who had arrived in England in 1939 from Budapest and set up a practice in his home in a Manchester suburb, Didsbury. He agreed to take Esther on for analysis for a minimal fee – 2s. a session – which she paid from her earnings in a job she now got teaching in a wartime day nursery in Salford. She loved it. 'It was very happy', she remembered, 'wonderful'. She was so keen for others to see exactly what went on that she told the staff, when the Queen visited, not to warn the mothers lest they dress their children in special clothes. She herself was very alert to what went on, including noticing the way in which the children's agitation and disturbance settled down when she gave them pebbles and empty cans into which to put them. It seemed she already intuitively knew of their need to be 'contained', as Bion later called this need in *Learning from Experience* (1962).

Perhaps it was the reputation Esther acquired through her work in the Salford nursery that led to her being asked to become a nursery adviser in Yorkshire's West Riding. Nurseries at that time were often staffed by women solely concerned to keep their charges outwardly clean and tidy. 'What they did with the children was terrible', she said: 'Babies they scrubbed and they washed them. In the mornings after breakfast they put them into chairs with strings to wait till lunchtime. And meanwhile they tore each other's hair out. It was so shocking'.[6] During the second half of the war, 1942–5, she worked as an adviser to put this situation right. She was also invited to work a couple of sessions a week treating children in a child guidance clinic in Leeds, for which she prepared herself by reading the books published by Anna Freud in 1927 and by Melanie Klein in 1932 about child analysis. She much preferred Klein's book. It was then, she later said, that she became a Kleinian.

When the war ended she moved back to London with Balint and another of his patients – a social worker, Betty Joseph. With Balint's encouragement they both applied for psychoanalytic training and were both accepted. Esther was supervised by James Strachey and Melanie Klein. Klein also supervised her treatment of her second adult training case, and her first child analysis case. With Balint's agreement Esther terminated her analysis with him and went into analysis with Klein, so impressed was she with Klein's lectures and teaching.

On first returning to London after the war she was again poverty-stricken. Betty helped her find work – one session a week doing psychological testing. She then got a child guidance job in Ealing. She enormously enjoyed it, especially her first case – a nine-year-old-boy whom she saw with his grandmother. She so much liked the job that she was unwilling to give it up for the work she was now invited to do at the Tavistock Clinic. But Balint persuaded her, and, in 1946, she started working there as a psychotherapist doing a couple of sessions a week for 2 guineas a session. In April 1948 she presented a clinical paper to the British Psycho-Analytical Society and the same year, now qualified as a psychoanalyst, and encouraged by John Bowlby, then Chair of the Tavistock's Children and Parents Department, she started the Tavistock's first child psychotherapy course. It was in this context that she first introduced infant observation as a means of teaching psychotherapy and other students about the inner world of children and adults.

Introducing infant observation

Bick's first child psychotherapy students in 1949 included Mary Boston, John Bremner and Yana Popper. The next year she herself qualified as a child analyst and added into her course a new group of trainees. They included Frances Tustin, Martha Harris and Dina Rosenbluth. Rosenbluth observed the twin baby sons of the psychoanalyst Sue Isaacs-Elmhirst, who later wrote about how Rosenbluth's observations evoked Bick's idealization of her mothering of them.[7] But it was objectivity Bick chiefly valued in infant observation. She maintained that, by observing babies in their first pre-clinical year of training, psychotherapy students acquire a particularly vivid understanding of the earliest experience patients bring with them into therapy. She encouraged students to find mothers and babies to observe through their GPs. She could be dogmatic about it. When one student, Joan Cornwall, recently arrived from Australia, said she had not yet got a GP, Bick insisted, 'But of course you have one'.[8]

Finding mothers to observe could be difficult. But they often proved happy to have someone visit for an hour a week for a couple of years from when their babies were first born. Bick also recommended that, so as to become maximally responsive to the mothers and babies they observed, students should not take notes while observing. Nor should they become too practically embroiled. Rather they should retain the warm and concerned detachment they would need as therapists.

Infant observation, she said, would also enable them to recover the feelings about early mothering that patients bring with them into therapy. In particular, she noted, observing mothers and babies helps familiarize students with the depression often afflicting mothers when their babies are first born. An example was a mother who, together with her husband, also in his mid-twenties, worked as an office caretaker. Two days after her son's birth, the observing student noted, the mother was radiant, but three days later she looked harassed and tired. She incessantly talked about having endlessly to feed and clean the baby, about how much it took to satisfy him, about a blister on her nipple, about pains under her arm. The student also noted sympathetically how, when her son cried, she seemed at a loss as to how to comfort him. Over the next weeks she evidently found it a terrible struggle trying to satisfy him – her 'wild, hungry baby'. When he screamed she either went on talking, apparently unconcerned, or she gave him to the student to hold and chatted on. Her husband helped. He gently indicated their son's feelings to her by imitating them. At the same time he made it clear he regarded her as the expert as far as their baby's care was concerned. As a result, and with time, she gradually became closer and more able to face and cope with his feelings.

Other students identify less with the mother than with the baby. An example, wrote Bick, was a student observing a professional couple and their baby, Charles. He described him at ten days: the 'motionless quality to his whole body as he sucked', his face afterwards looking 'calm but rather bloated and expressionless'. He also described Charles crying 'miserably' as he was changed, his hands constantly around his face, his left hand moving in front of him with a stroking action as though he were a 'blind man'. He described Charles falling asleep, occasionally half waking, puckering and crying at noises from his nineteen-month-old brother's room. Later the student noted that, when Charles had been lying on the cot mattress while his mother and grandmother busied themselves collecting things for a walk, his expression on awaking was 'fixed in a look of great pain of an intense kind, and not a muscle moved for the two or three minutes between when I first saw it and when I said goodbye to them outside the house'.[9]

Bick also quoted her students' observations to highlight the different sensory modalities through which babies and mothers relate to each other. Some, she noted, relate mainly through sight and sound. This was the case, for instance, with the baby son of a Mrs A. After feeding him, she put him on the floor or held him apart from her body as she looked at him. She made movements and sounds with her lips as she did so, to which he responded in like fashion. It was seeing and hearing her that he most missed when she was out of the room. All then went well, the student noted, provided he held him on his lap without reminding him of his mother's absence by talking or looking at him.

Other babies relate less through talking and looking than through holding and touching. One baby, for instance, avoided both holding and touching when he was not on his mother's lap but the student's. With his mother, by contrast, it was all holding and touching. When she put him to the breast he immediately latched on and sucked vigorously, eyes open, his right hand alternately touching her breast and the button on her dress. At thirteen weeks it was the same: he felt for her breast with his mouth and hand and then used his hand to hold on to her arm. It was the same after his bath: he clutched at her breast, put his hand on top of hers and moved it rhythmically as he too moved. It was the same when, initially protesting at being weaned at twenty-seven weeks, he was fed by her with a bottle. He touched it, reached out for it, lovingly stroked it, and, keeping one hand on the bottle, used the other to touch, stroke and caress her.

One student described Bick's remarkable capacity for bringing the personalities of babies alive as manifesting a 'poetic quality displayed only by those who love life intensely'.[10] Poetic or not, she certainly stressed the importance of choosing the right words. Determining their rightness, she said, depends on testing one observation against the next. It also depends on trainees discussing and comparing with their fellow students their successive observations. Getting together to talk about their observations, she maintained, also helps students cope with differences between mothers and babies and their idiosyncrasies in the way they learn to relate to each other.

As an example of one such mother–baby couple, and of putting together successive observations, Bick returned to Charles (see p. 140 above). At ten days he was more frantic at the first breast, whereas at the second breast he patted it, formed a trumpet shape with his hand around his mouth, sucking very gently and slowly. Subsequently, left alone, his hand again made a trumpet shape and he fell asleep. The same pattern of initial excitement at the first breast followed by calm at the second continued in subsequent observations through his first three months. By ten weeks he regularly fed at the first breast with his hand on his mother's chest, his fingers sometimes clenching or with both hands on either side of the breast, motionless. This was followed at the second breast by his gently stroking and caressing it.

Charles constituted the final example in Bick's first and only published account of her infant observation approach to psychotherapy and psychoanalytic training. She concluded by reiterating its value in strengthening student recognition of the early mothering that patients bring within them into therapy. It was a theme to which she also returned in an essay she wrote in 1953 for membership of the British Psycho-Analytic Society. In it she also introduced an idea to which she returned again and again over the next thirty years: the way in which, in the absence of feeling protectively mothered and contained inside, children and adults may cling for comfort to an outer surface or skin.

Outer clinging

In her essay of 1953 Bick illustrated the point with the example of a married woman she first began treating in 1948.[11] Born in 1916, the patient arrived in analysis complaining of claustrophobic fear of being trapped in underground trains and theatres, of being hemmed in by crowds, and of terror of suffocating when she pulled her clothes on over her head or washed her hair. She was also terrified of sex, and had never had intercourse with her husband. She was too small, she said, it would shatter her inside.

These terrors, it turned out, were linked to the upset of her mother suddenly dying five years before, when the patient was briefly away from home. But her fears were most of all linked to an image of herself as being tiny, like a baby clinging with her mouth to her husband as though she were a vampire or leech. Her terror that vampire-like clinging would destroy those she loved paralysed her. She looked to Bick to protect her from herself in the absence of any inner sense of having been protected by her mother as a baby, because at that time her mother had been so preoccupied with, and depressed by, her husband being called up to fight at the front in the First World War. Bick's patient also protected herself by imagining it was not her but others who sucked and clung like vampires. It was this that made her fearful of being trapped and suffocated, and of being shattered by sex. Gradually, however, through Bick helping her recover more than a fraction of protective early mothering she initially brought with her into analysis, her fears and symptoms decreased, and she became more hopeful of enjoying sex.

Bick saw this woman and other patients in the late 1940s and early 1950s in a consulting-room in her flat in 16 Kent Terrace, near Regent's Park. Subsequently she moved to a third-floor flat in 4 Compayne Mansions in West Hampstead. The flat had a beautiful turretted living-room. But Bick's hardships continued. The rest of her home was a slum. There was an old stone sink and a tap held together with wire in the kitchen; lino in patches on the floors; everything in a generally dilapidated condition. It was different with psychoanalysis. Bick devoted her all to it – and to Israel, where she discovered her brother had settled and had a daughter, Zvia. Bick shared her involvement in Israel with one of her early child psychotherapy students, Isca Wittenberg. Wittenberg also recalls from her infant observation training, beginning in 1956, Bick's 'great capacity to be in touch with and convey the baby's experience'.[12]

Bick was less in touch with the experience of her Tavistock colleagues and with the need to be diplomatic with them. They became increasingly critical of her narrowly Kleinian views. But she refused to compromise and in 1959 Bowlby told her he would no longer be asking her to run the child psychotherapy course she had started. She continued to teach and supervise its students, but from 1960 the course itself was run by one of her first students – Martha ('Mattie') Harris.[13] Earlier that summer Bick fetched Klein home from Switzerland when she became very ill on holiday there, and, soon after Klein's death that autumn, the London Institute of Psycho-Analysis introduced Bick's infant observation method into its training programme. Or, at least, it introduced what she regarded as a very 'watered down', one-year version of her method.

The next August Bick spoke in Edinburgh about child analysis at the first symposium devoted to the subject by a psychoanalytic congress.[14] But it is for her infant observation essay of 1964 that she is now best known. Within psychoanalysis she is also known for her subsequent account of the outer clinging of children and adults in defence against inner lack of integration. She spoke about this to the congress in Copenhagen held in July 1967. She began her talk by noting the initial lack of integration of babies and the way they look to something outside – a light, a voice, a smell – to bring them together. In the first instance, she noted, babies are brought together by being held and surrounded by the smell, talk and physical and emotional presence of their mothers feeding them. Taking into themselves the feeling of being held and contained within their mothers' arms and minds, babies feel held together in their skin.

Bick illustrated the point with a student's observation of a baby girl whose initial lack of integration was evident in her trembling, sneezing and disorganized movements. Over the next few weeks, however, thanks to her taking in her mother's increasing closeness with her, the little girl became more integrated. But this was disrupted when she was twelve weeks old and the family moved home. Her mother now became more distant, watched TV while she fed her and at night fed her in the dark, without holding her. She withdrew still more when her husband became ill. Then she became preoccupied with getting a job. To all this, her baby daughter, feeling starved of being held by her mother, lost her previously precariously achieved sense of being held together. Her lack of integration spilled out in bodily ills and she was held together only by developing a brittle outer shell. Bick called it a 'second skin', and described it in this little girl's case as involving pseudo-independence, aggression and pummelling people's faces, cheered on by her mother praising her as a 'boxer'.

A similar process occurred in one of Bick's child analysis cases, Mary, who, from Bick's account of the case, was probably the daughter of Ann and Adrian Stokes, Ariadne.[15] Bick described her as 'schizophrenic' and as first coming into analysis when she was three and a half. Her lack of integration at that time, said Bick, included her starting sessions by emitting an explosive 'SSBICK' for 'Good morning, Mrs Bick'. Her lack of integration was also evident, Bick added, in her body being hunched, stiff-jointed, grotesque, like a 'sack of potatoes', as Mary herself later put it, and as Adrian Stokes put it in a poem to his daughter (see p. 88 above). With analysis, however, there was some slight improvement. The precarious outer 'sack' gave way to Mary feeling contained within her skin, within her own 'muscularity', as Bick put it.

Other clinical examples of sack-like outer holding and containing included a man who held himself together through constantly looking to others to praise him. Another example was a five-year-old, Jill, who held herself together with the outer reassurance of having her clothes firmly fastened and her shoes tightly laced. Otherwise she feared breaking into pieces just as toys break, she told Bick, because 'Toys are not like me . . . They don't have a skin'.[16]

Bick went on in subsequent teaching and seminars to describe how some children and adults avert not feeling securely held together inside by recourse to a sort of sticky outer clinging. 'I don't know how to talk about it', she told her psychoanalyst colleague Donald Meltzer (then married to her successor in running the Tavistock child psychotherapy course that she had founded). 'They are just like that', she said, putting her hands together, 'They stick'.[17]

Mary was a case in point. Her lack of integration on first seeing Bick included a streaming nose, lack of toilet-training and uncontrolled movements. She later described herself then as 'spilling out'. At first she fended it off by clinging to Bick and by quickly becoming very attached to her. She called her 'Choki Biki' and became as if physically attached to her. She stuck to Bick's words. She parroted and repeated them. She also became stuck to her chair: at the end of their sessions together she could not get up out of it. When at last she managed to stand up and move she would become stuck to the door knob, turning it round and round, unable to leave. She clung to Bick, just as she clung to her mother to avert terror of lacking integration, as Bick put it, of lacerating separation, of what Mary called 'spilling out'.

Another child, Sonia, who like Mary also suffered severe retardation, and who was referred for analysis when she was six and a half, expressed similar sticky clinging. Bick called it 'adhesive identification'. One session she drew two clinging or joining loops which she went on looping, one after another. Then, after the weekend break, she started the next session by getting up on the furniture and looping along the wall until she got to the highest point, scratched the ceiling and said of the plaster that then fell to the floor: 'That is to stop the gap'. At the end of sessions she often stopped the gap by lying on the sink, putting her mouth to the tap, filling her mouth with water and holding onto the water in her mouth until her mother came into sight. Only then did she swallow the water which she then replaced by holding onto her mother with her eyes. Another time she wrote the letter 'J', standing for 'Jew', for her being different from others in being handicapped. When she came to the end of the letter – the 'dead-end', as she called it – she stopped the gap by going on drawing, round and round.

Among Bick's other patients were Mrs B, who described the 'gap' or 'dead-end' as a space she dreaded falling into from her surface-level, two-dimensional 'flat earth' world; and Mrs S, who brought a dream one Thursday of the fourth of five lambs crying to the fifth that he would die on the Friday, before the weekend break, unless he listened closely to Mrs Bick reading a book. Safety lay in clinging to her words. As her analysis progressed, Mrs S felt more held together and contained by her treatment. She was more able to find words inside. She compared herself to a centipede holding on with a hundred feet. 'Only', she added, drawing on what she retained within her from childhood, 'in my country it is called a millepede'.[18]

Infant observation provides similar examples. One was a baby who averted lack of integration – evident, said Bick, in his quivering and shaking on having his clothes taken off for a bath – by clinging to the outer sensation of his mother touching him with wet cotton wool. At other times he clung, as it were, with his ears to the continuous sound of the washing machine. For another baby initial lack of integration was evident in his hands and arms flying out when his mother laid him on her lap as though, wrote the student observing him, he were an 'astronaut in a gravity-less zone'. But then his mother brought him together. She gently talked to him, held his hands together with hers, and, as she changed him, talked understandingly of how he disliked it.

In England, Bick taught students from the Commonwealth, the USA and France; she also travelled to teach in South America, Spain, Switzerland and Italy. While in Italy in 1972, the year of a large Henry Moore exhibition, she holidayed in Florence with her Kleinian friends Elinor and Claude Wedeles (with whom she had also stayed in the 1960s in their country home on Clough Williams Ellis's estate in North Wales). On arriving in Florence she told the Wedeles that Adrian Stokes had said there was nothing to see there,[19] that Venice was the only place.

Back in London she held infant observation seminars in her home and in that of the Wedeleses at 13 Eton Road. Between 1972 and 1977 her seminars included a fortnightly meeting with other psychoanalysts, including Donald Meltzer, Elizabeth Bott-Spillius and Elinor Wedeles. As with her students, she insisted that her colleagues always provide detailed reports. 'She'd hit the roof', Wedeles recalls, 'if one suggested simply summarising one's observations'. The same quality characterized the seminar she began running for experienced child psychotherapists in 1979 (and continued to run after her retirement as an analyst in 1980). She wanted every little detail, wrote one of the seminar's members, Jeanne Magagna, so 'she could experience with Proustian clarity the relationship between the baby and his family'.[20]

Magagna also drew attention to Bick's account of the baby's fear of disintegration. Bick herself was now beginning to disintegrate. In her late seventies she began to lose her memory, her health failed, and she was briefly hospitalized because of a kidney problem. It led to her moving to a room in Campden Hill Square and then to a nursing home, found for her by Betty Joseph in Redbridge on the Essex outskirts of London. She was now becoming increasingly mentally infirm. Nevertheless, Mattie Harris observed, her nurses were fascinated by her life story. But she was not with them long. She died on 20 July 1983, leaving a legacy of infant observation training and insights about flight from inner lack of integration to outer clinging – insights developed particularly illuminatingly by Frances Tustin.

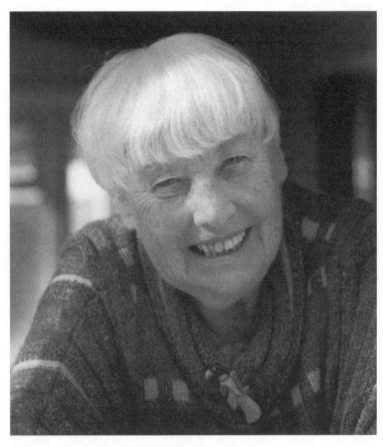

Frances Tustin, 1990/1

8 Frances Tustin: Anorexia and Autism

Bion's widow, Francesca, recalls Frances Tustin as 'exceptional'. She was particularly exceptional, as a therapist, in overturning the still prevalent dogma that autism is untreatable. In doing so, Tustin drew on what she learnt from successfully treating autistic and anorexic children, and on what they taught her about their own experience, about that of others she treated, and about herself and her early closeness with her mother.

Early closeness[1]

Frances's mother was very religious. She was educated at Chelsea College in London and became a deaconess in the Church of England. It was through the church, in which she was known as 'Sister Minnie', that she first met her husband, George Vickers. He was fourteen years younger than Minnie and had trained as a lay reader in the Church Army. Not long after Frances's birth – in Darlington on 13 October 1913 – he was sent abroad, following the outbreak of war, to serve as an army chaplain in France, where he was taken prisoner. Frances grew up for the next five years alone with her mother in what Sheila Spensley described as an 'atmosphere of smothering devotion to the Church's teaching'.[2] Frances later described herself in this period as an enthusiastic member of the Church's Band of Hope, convinced of being a 'sunbeam for Jesus' lighting a world of 'darkness and sin'.[3] She also recalled being brought up to be a little 'sister' to her mother. This included guiding her mother through the streets in the black-out

because she was smaller and nearer the pavement and could therefore see it better.

When at last her father came home he had lost the faith that had
first brought him and her mother together. Deeply disillusioned by
the Church's attitudes to the war, he had become a pacifist and a
socialist. On leaving the army, he took the family to Scotland, where
they lived for a short while before settling in Sheffield. It was there
that Frances began school and her father went to university to study
to become a teacher. Minnie was totally against his going to university: she was convinced it would infect him with the devil. In their
resulting conflict Frances sided with her father, and rejected her
mother's beliefs as superstitious, narrow-minded dogma. She preferred her father's spirit of freedom, which led him, among other
things, to take her for a week to Summerhill, the progressive school
started in 1921 in Suffolk by A. S. Neill, an analysand of Wilhelm
Reich, whose ideas, along with those of Freud, Frances's mother
condemned as wicked and evil.

But for Minnie's opposition George might have got a teaching job
at Summerhill but instead, after completing his teacher training, he
worked in a number of country schools in Lincolnshire. Soon he
became headmaster of a village school which Frances also attended.
She loved the country, but Minnie hated it, being frightened of cows,
dogs and the dark. She much preferred the life of the town, symbolically suggesting this through her penchant for wearing white evening
gloves. She disapproved of her husband's country-loving ways – his
cloth cap and his love of his family's Lincolnshire farming background, a background that included among his forebears the Quaker
prison reformer Elizabeth Fry and the first woman preacher, the
Wesleyan Sarah Crisp.

With all the tension between her parents Frances was glad to
get away: aged twelve, she won a scholarship to Sleaford High
School, where she had to board because her home was too far from
the station for her to get there each day by train. Within a year,
however, her father got a job in another village school from which
Frances could become a day-pupil at Grantham High School. She
transferred there and was put in the scholarship stream with
hopes of eventually going to Oxford to study biology. But it was
not to be.

When Frances was thirteen her mother decided to leave her
husband and to take their daughter with her. This decision came as
a complete shock to Frances. She wondered how she could hide so
as not to be torn away. But torn away she was and the two of them
spent the next year travelling around England, living with friends
and relatives, before returning to Sheffield, where Minnie took a job

working in a small, rather run-down church. It left them poverty-stricken. Opposing free-thinking in the name of her religion, Minnie used Frances's grammar school scholarship to transfer her to a school that would prepare her to become a teacher. In 1932 she was sent to Whitelands in Putney, where she trained to become a junior school teacher specializing in biology. Years later she remembered enjoying Whitelands and its evening service words, 'I shall repose upon thy eternal changelessness'. It was a High Anglican college but progressive. Its founders included John Ruskin, and its staff during Frances's time there followed the liberal educational philosophy of Homer Lane, championing children's freedom, love and self-government.

On graduating Frances returned to Sheffield to be near her mother, whose health was now failing. But she also distanced herself from her in becoming a socialist like her father. Through the Sheffield Labour Party she met John Taylor, a Town Hall official, whom she married in 1938, but from whom she was soon separated when, following the outbreak of the Second World War, he was called up. After her mother's death in 1942 Frances was able to leave Sheffield to work in a progressive boarding school in Kent, from which she travelled to attend Susan Isaacs's London-based child development course in the evenings.

As for the progressive school, Frances was very taken with its freedom from dogma: it minimized rules that might cause the children feelings of guilt, rejection or lack of self-esteem; it provided self-governing meetings for the children; it encouraged pupils and teachers to address each other equally by their first names; and it instituted project work, enabling the children to pursue what interested them most. Among the projects Frances introduced was one described by Marion Milner in *An Experiment in Leisure* (1937) and by Herbert Read in *Education through Art* (1943). Taking her cue from Milner and Read, she suggested to the twelve children in the group for which she was responsible that they close their eyes and watch for visual images – 'mind-pictures', she called them – flashing before their eyes. The children, aged between seven and ten, were very taken with this exercise. One of the nine-year-olds exclaimed, 'I've got a lovely idea. I'll do a "head" and what the head is thinking', whereupon he drew a tramp, with a picture in the tramp's head. In her book *A Group of Juniors* (1951) Frances described it as 'exactly the kind of wish-fulfilment picture such a deprived person is likely to have . . . a neat house with a trim garden and a big cheery sun in the sky . . . [with] a woman in a full skirt to welcome [him]'.[4] It was akin perhaps to her own thoughts when, aged thirteen, she had, as it were, tramped around England with her mother.

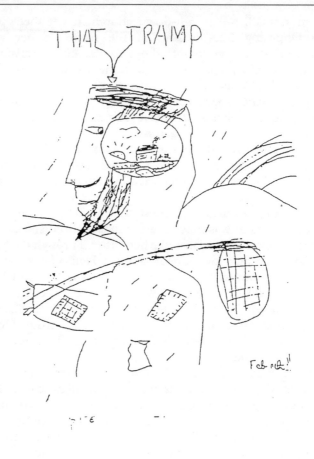

Mind-picture of a tramp

Frances's work with these children ended after the war. When her husband returned, they found they had grown apart and decided to separate: John returned to Sheffield and Frances got a lecturing job in 1946 at her old college, Whitelands. She also became increasingly involved with Arnold Tustin, who was married and fourteen years her senior. They had first met in 1942 through a liberal Christian group, Commonwealth. He was a pioneer in cybernetics, including studying circuits in the brain which Frances related to her work with children. More immediately she helped nurse him back to health when he became very ill following surgery at the time of his divorce in 1946 from his first wife, Frieda. Soon after, and with Frances's encouragement, he applied for a professorship in electrical engineering at Birmingham University, to which he was appointed in 1947. The next year they married and Frances got another lecturing job, this time in a Birmingham teacher training college in Dudley near Edgbaston where she and Arnold settled in 37 Carpenter Road.

Around this time she also rediscovered her father – through a letter he had written to *The Times* – but she was disappointed, in meeting him again, that he was as hostile to his new wife, Gladys, as he had been to her mother. She was also disappointed later by his giving up the anarchism of his younger days and becoming a Roman Catholic. Meanwhile, on first marrying, she and Arnold rented out the top floor of their Carpenter Road home to one of Arnold's colleagues, David Munrow, and his wife, Hilda. The Munrows' son, David (later an eminent early music specialist), became something of a substitute child to Frances when, in 1949, she suffered toxaemia of pregnancy and lost the baby she was carrying. She was grief-stricken. Having been interested in psychoanalysis since reading Marion Milner's *An Experiment in Leisure* (1937), and encouraged by a Tavistock-based psychoanalyst, Dugmore Hunter, whom she met through her work on *A Group of Juniors*, she decided to train in child psychotherapy. In 1950 she began Esther Bick's Tavistock course, and stayed in London during the week with her fellow student Mattie Harris and her husband, Roland.

Initially she had misgivings about Bick and her dogmatic Kleinianism. She also had misgivings about Bion, to whom Bick recommended her for analysis. She found him forbidding and dominating. Of their first meeting she later wrote: 'I thought, "This is terrible". The great bushy eyebrows and those stern eyes. I wondered what I'd come to. It felt as if he just took me and flung me on the couch. I was really quite frightened by him, I think. There were a lot of silences which I always hated'.[5] But she was soon won over. He was so 'rare', she recalled, both 'awful' and 'awesome'.[6] Apart from a break when she was in the US, and another when she suffered a second miscarriage, she remained in analysis with him for fourteen years.

While at the Tavistock she was supervised by Herbert Rosenfeld and Donald Meltzer. It was now that she also first became interested in autism, in part through Marion Putnam's account of the work with autistic children of the Putnam Center in Boston, given at the Tavistock in 1952. With John Bowlby's encouragement she applied to work as a therapist at the centre while Arnold held a year's visiting Webster Professorship (1954–5) at the nearby Massachusetts Institute of Technology. While at the centre she provided respite care for parents and learnt first-hand of their plight when she was faced with their autistic children's unresponsiveness. Her work in Boston also acquainted her with the theories of the psychoanalyst Margaret Mahler, who located the origins of childhood schizophrenia in what Mahler maintained is every child's initial 'symbiotic' oneness with its mother.

Frances continued working with autistic children on returning to England when Arnold was appointed to a chair at the University of London's Imperial College in Kensington. They settled nearby first in Thurloe Square, and then in 57 Palace Gardens Terrace, where Frances established her consulting-room. She also worked at Great Ormond Street Children's Hospital with Mildred Creak, a specialist in childhood psychosis and autism.

Anorexia

While working with the psychoanalyst Sydney Klein at the West Middlesex Hospital in 1955, Frances Tustin saw the patient who became the subject of her first published case history – about anorexia. The case concerned a teenager, Margaret.[7] Margaret weighed less than 4 stone when, aged thirteen, she was first seen in the hospital's paediatrics department on 16 November 1955. No organic cause could be found for her weight loss, so she was referred to the psychiatric department where, because she was so emaciated, she was admitted as an in-patient. Her mother said she had first begun losing weight on returning to school that September, when she said she had to get thin for a ballet exam she was due to take a couple of months later. She had virtually stopped eating. She also fainted when her class was shown a sex education film. Seeing blood, she said, made her sick. She did not want to know about it, or about menstruation. But she was intensely interested in her aunt's pregnancy and in that of a neighbour.

Margaret was born in 1942, while her father was away in the war in the navy. When she was four months old her mother was so upset on learning his ship had gone missing that her milk stopped. Despite learning three months later that he was alive and well, she remained depressed and, when Margaret was two, she also became diabetic. On his return she became pregnant, at which Margaret became so ill with gastro-enteritis she had to be hospitalized. Soon afterwards her brother, Robin, was born, and subseqeuntly two more boys. Margaret's father openly said he preferred boys to girls. It threw Margaret together with her mother, who said they had a very close relationship: Margaret was like a younger sister with whom she could share everything, including her early wish to become a dancer.

On first meeting Margaret in the hospital on 9 January 1956, Tustin explained she should say whatever came into her mind so they could try to understand why she did not want to eat. At first Margaret was uneasy. She said nothing. Perhaps she was uneasy, Tustin suggested, at meeting yet another stranger. But Margaret remained mute. Eventually, after a long pause, she whispered haltingly and so softly that Tustin had to lean close to hear, that her teacher had been supposed to come that morning but had not arrived. Tustin commented that Margaret feared Tustin too would raise her hopes only to disappoint them. But Tustin assured her she would see her for half an hour every Monday, Tuesday and Friday morning. At this Margaret, who was curled up under a blanket and looked like a baby, said she had put on weight. She continued putting on weight over the next two weeks – as long as she felt that, as with her mother, she and Tustin shared everything, including what she saw as Tustin's life-giving energy and power.

But this honeymoon sharing soon ended. It was succeeded by her experiencing Tustin as separate, free and pretty – as utterly different from her experience of herself as dowdy and inhibited. She envied and hated Tustin for being different. She worried Tustin might similarly hate her. She thought that was why Tustin did not see her more often and that Tustin wanted to stop her growing up to become a woman like her. With this she again lost weight and continued to do so when her aunt came into hospital to have her baby. Again she suffered gastro-enteritis, as she had when her mother was pregnant with her brother Robin.

At first Margaret put on weight only while she imagined that she and Tustin were the same. She imagined they were both pregnant. But when this phantasy collapsed she imagined that in putting on weight she was becoming pregnant at Tustin's expense. She felt she drained and exhausted Tustin and had lost her good will. She despaired of ever recovering Tustin's interest in her just as, when she was a baby, she despaired of ever recovering her mother's interest in her when her mother was depressed and ill with diabetes. The only thing that pleased her mother then was jiggling her on her knee. That was why she wanted to become a dancer, in the hope that this too would please her mother. She dreaded failing. That was why she got ill – to get out of doing the dancing exam lest she fail it. That was why she did not want to know about blood or menstruation. It meant becoming a woman, thereby putting an end to her mother's longing for her to have been a boy. She also feared menstruation because the blood seemed to signify the damage done by her hating and envying her mother as separate and different from her.

In exploring these issues Margaret oscillated between eating and not eating depending on whether she felt the same or different from Tustin. Gradually, however, her weight gain became more sustained. By the end of March 1957, two and half months after her treatment began, she had improved sufficiently to go home. She continued seeing Tustin as an out-patient and went on getting better as she became increasingly able to express issues of sameness and difference less outwardly, through what she ate and weighed, and more inwardly, through what she thought and felt. By April 1957 she was so much better that she could return to school and, on leaving, got a job. She reduced therapy to once a week, managed a long break (when Tustin was ill for many months following her second miscarriage), and also coped with resuming her therapy after Tustin recovered, even though this meant travelling a long way by bus to Tustin's Kensington consulting-room.

In understanding her case Tustin drew on what she had learnt at the Tavistock about Klein's theory of depression. She also drew perhaps on what she knew from her closeness with her own mother when she too was thirteen and lived alone with her on their leaving her father. Arguably she also drew on what she had learnt from her work at the Putnam Center and Mahler's theory about children's initial closeness with and subsequent individuating separateness from their mothers. Klein was annoyed with Frances's resulting departure from her theories, at which Arnold Tustin expostulated, 'The stupid woman! Of course it is not her work. It is your work!'[8]

Drawing, perhaps, on what she had learnt from treating Margaret, Frances wrote more about issues of sameness and difference, closeness and separation, in her next published case history. It too concerned a child with eating difficulties – a nine-year-old boy called Paul who first came into therapy when he was six and a half, both because of his resistance to eating and because he so hated being separated from his parents that he refused to go to school.[9] All went well, provided he imagined he and his parents were the same. All likewise went well in his therapy, provided he felt Tustin conformed with his expectation that she would go along with everything he wanted. Faced with difference and separation from her, however, he became enraged. He drew people with thought-bubbles coming out of their heads full of mocking and teasing words. He drew pictures of rat-like animals eroding the ground, of birds of prey feeding on dead bodies, and of ice creams whisked away just as a man was about to eat them.

Paul drew wild lions and lions in cages. After a ten-day break in his therapy, he drew another lion. As he drew it he said he had read that lions attack only if they are hungry, disturbed or if their cubs are threatened. He had eaten only a little during the break, he added as he drew a leash on the lion to hold it back from eating a joint of raw meat. It was his drawing of the same lion shape after another break in his therapy that alerted Tustin to the significance of his previous picture. He drew the route taking him from his house to her con-sulting-room. As he drew it he emphasized that the point corre-sponding to the eye of the lion marked the spot where there was a butcher's shop. It seemed Tustin had become meat in his mind, into which he so wanted to tear during the break that he had to hold himself back – hence the leash (see next page).

Paul's case led Tustin to understand autism in a new light – as an effect of rage at separation being so great that it cannot even be contemplated, so much is it equated with tearing into, bodily wrench-ing apart, thus leaving a hole into which biting rage, represented as monsters, threatens to rush back.

Black hole depression

It was in the terms of Paul's case that Tustin now recounted her treatment in the early 1950s of an autistic boy, John, who taught her about the depressing terror of what he called a 'black hole'. At one of Tustin's talks someone in the audience linked John's 'black hole' with Winnicott's theory of primary depression, involving babies experiencing maternal separation as equivalent to losing part of their bodies. Winnicott's theory was news to Tustin, she later wrote. It had been excluded as 'misguided' from the Kleinianism she had been taught by Bick at the Tavistock when she was first treating John.[10] Writing up his case over ten years later, however, she openly drew on Winnicott's theories, as well as on those of Klein and Mahler.

Tustin described John as first being referred for psychiatric treat-ment when he was two and a half because he still had no speech and was generally very retarded.[11] The psychiatrist thought he might be mentally defective because of the way he held a toy car upside down to spin its wheels. Six months later he was more optimistic when John played with cars the right way up. He referred him to Mildred Creak, who diagnosed possible autism. Hopeful that John's seeking to make contact with her by touching her hand boded well for therapy, Creak in turn referred the child to Tustin.

John's father had a schizophrenic sister. As a result of her father having died when she was still a child, John's mother had mostly been brought up in an institution. She had been impatient to grow up, and was similarly impatient for John to grow up. She had spent her childhood in a remote village in Scotland, and was upset by the

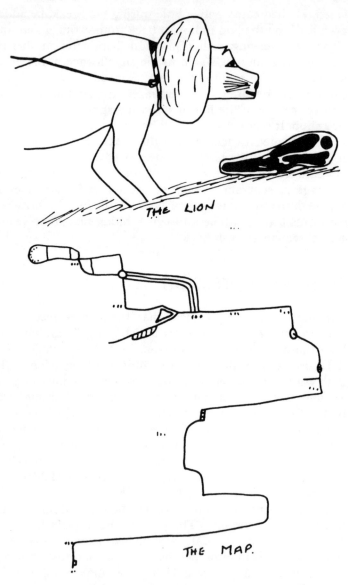

Paul's lion and map pictures

foreign-seeming procedures of the maternity hospital in England where John was born. This was compounded by John not opening his eyes for the first week after his birth, by his sucking so poorly she could not breastfeed him, and by their having to stay with her sister-in-law on leaving the maternity hospital because John's father was away working in another town.

Eighteen months later they had another child – a little girl. John showed little reaction. But what worried his parents most was his lack of speech, and his strange behaviour: his bizarre hand movements, in which he moved his fingers in front of his face in a strange, stiff way; his lack of response to people; and his not playing with other children on the roundabout in the park, for instance. He was more interested in looking under it to see how it worked. His parents were also worried by his refusing to eat anything but soft food, and by his lack of bladder and bowel control.

In November 1951, when he was three and a half, he started seeing Tustin for therapy, at first once a week, then three times, and eventually five times a week. At first he treated her as though she did not exist. He walked straight past her and ignored her, except to pull her hand to a humming-top to get her to spin it for him. As she spun it he became very flushed, leant forward to watch it spin, spun his penis through his trouser pocket, and at the same time spun his other hand around his mouth.

At his second meeting with Tustin, and again and again subsequently, he played with the humming-top. Eventually Tustin commented that he used his hand to spin the 'Tustin top', as she called it, so he could feel they were the same, that he was her and she was him, that they would always be together. At this he took a mummy doll and spun the bead holding a handbag to her hand, just as he spun his penis when Tustin spun the top. He then tapped the mummy doll, threw it to the ground and said 'Gone'. It was the first word Tustin had ever heard him say.

Verbalizing his fear of making his mummy gone led to further progress. John began facing his fear of difference and separation. This became particularly evident in one session, for instance, when, faced with Tustin refusing to do his bidding, he violently took her hand – as though it were a joined-on appendage of his own – to make the top spin. Then he spat and threw the top at the ceiling; it crashed to the ground, its insides falling out as it broke into two pieces. This made John utterly miserable. He went over to the top, saying 'Broken!' and 'Oh dear!', and spent the rest of the session hopelessly trying to mend it.

A similar sequence of tantrums and misery occurred after the Easter break when his father was away. He obsessively tapped a button on a cushion in Tustin's consulting-room, saying 'Daddy! Daddy!' as he did so. He had tantrums when he realized the button, and a toy he called the 'red Daddy bus' were not part of him and would not always do what he wanted. He followed his tantrums with dolefully saying, 'Broken! Gone! Oh dear!'

The idea of things being broken and gone led to John's at last saying 'I', a year after his treatment began. His father was back home and brought him to one of his sessions in November 1952. But at Tustin's doorstep he tripped and nearly fell down, whereupon John spent the ensuing session jumping up and down on the couch saying, 'Daddy mended! Daddy mended!' But when he found his father was not there to fetch him at the end of the session, that his mother had come to fetch him instead, he was panic-stricken. He screamed, 'Daddy! Daddy gone! Daddy broken!' In the night he woke yelling. It was then that he first used the personal pronoun 'I', screaming 'I don't want it! Fell down! Button broken! Don't let it bite! Don't let it bump!'

The button figured both in his night-time screaming and in his therapy. One session two months later, after seeing a baby being breastfed, he arranged four coloured pencils in the shape of a cross. As he did so he touched his mouth, saying, 'Breast!' and 'Button in the middle!' Then he put more pencils on the cross saying, 'Make a bigger breast! Make a bigger breast!' Tustin commented that he wanted a bigger breast than was actually there. At this he angrily knocked the pencils apart saying, 'Broken breast!' Then he added, 'I fix it! I fix it! Hole gone! Button on! Hole gone! Button on!'

As his therapy progressed he became increasingly able to face things being gone. He also became more able to face his dependence on Tustin as a separate figure to whom, when things were beyond his control, he appealed saying, 'I can't do it! Please help me!' Following a longer than usual break in his treatment, when he also had to stay away from home with his grandparents and had further night-time screaming fits, he regressed. But now he was more able to talk about the terrors involved. They included hallucinations of birds about to peck him.

John would also talk about his terrors in his play. Just over a year into his treatment, in January 1954, he again arranged some pencils into what he called a breast and, touching his mouth as he did so, said, 'Button in the middle!' Then he stood a pencil in the middle saying, 'Rocket!' He called the whole thing a 'firework breast'. It was linked to a drawing he had previously done of a dome-shaped object with brown and red 'stinkers' coming out. He called them 'fireworks'. Now, holding his mouth as if it hurt, he said, 'Prick in my mouth!' Then he said, 'Falls down! Button broken! Nasty black hole in my mouth!' Then, holding his penis, he said, 'Pee-pee still here?', as if it might have gone.

To all this Tustin explained that he felt the button – the breast – was part of his mouth. When he discovered they were separate it made him furious. His fury left a black hole into which he dreaded his fury and rage might rush back as though they were birds threat-

ening to peck him, or fireworks, a rocket, a prick in the mouth. Taking
in John's fury, understanding it, and helping him put the accompanying terrors into words, Tustin enabled him increasingly to face difference and separation between them. By July 1954, when he was six
and a half, he was so much better that he coped without therapy and
attended a normal school, where he was quick to learn and verbally
well in advance of his fellow pupils; he went on to public school and
university.

John had begun therapy clinging to outer things and shapes – to
toy cars and to the humming-top. Two years after his case was published, Bick's account of such clinging in terms of escape from lack
of inner integration appeared.[12] Tustin now added this to her understanding of autism helped by what she had learnt from another child
whom she characterized as 'encapsulated'.

Autistic encapsulation

Tustin called the patient involved David.[13] She described him as
always arriving at his therapy (four times a week) clinging so tightly
to a dinky car that it left a deep shape etched into his hand. He
equated the car – an Aston Martin – with the name of his family's
village home, Martin, and with Tustin's name. The words had the
same shape. That was what mattered: the outer sensation, not their
meaning or function. He was very withdrawn and used speech only
to relieve tension, not to relate to other people. He could not learn
at school. He greeted frustration with rage. And he could not be
trusted outdoors because he was so heedless of danger.

David's mother had been bitterly disappointed at his birth – at his
being a boy. Already having one boy, she wanted a girl. She was also
disappointed at his having a twisted spine – a disability similar to one
his father suffered. To get it treated she weaned David when he was
five months old so he could stay in a 'Baby Hotel' in London and
see a masseuse, with whom he continued treatment until he was thirteen months old, when the masseuse said he would do better being
with his family at home. When he was five he started infant school,
but he proved unteachable, and was sent first to a Rudolf Steiner
school and then to a small boarding school in Hampstead. Here the
teacher, Mrs Fiona, suspecting his difficulties were emotional,
arranged for him to be referred to the Tavistock Clinic; aged ten and
a half, all he would do for the assessing psychologist there was draw
a ruined house.

His therapy with Tustin began soon after. Four years later he was
sufficiently recovered to travel on his own from Hampstead to see

her in Kensington. Tustin described two sessions from this period in his therapy. The first occurred just before a half-term break. He arrived preoccupied with a boil on the second finger of his right hand. He said the boil was a 'monster', talked about 'boiling with rage', asked about a 'boiler' in the passage outside her consulting-room, saying 'It might explode like a volcano'. Then he said his teacher, Mrs Fiona, had squeezed the boil and 'nasty pus had spurted out'. He called it 'lava' and 'death juice', to which he added, 'There's a hole all blocked up with gritty bits of dead skin where the boil has gone'.

Later he linked a ball in the drawer where Tustin kept his things with the boil saying, 'This ball – this boil – did you hear what I said? This ball/boil'. Then the ball rolled under the couch. He retrieved it saying, 'Naughty thing! It's gone! Why did it go under there?' Addressing the ball, he ordered it, 'You stay in my hands', adding, 'This thing full of gas! I will trap and squeeze it and it will go off pop!' Then he said, 'When the tits are busted they leave gritty bits of dead skin'.

They were all linked together – the half-term break, tits being busted and gone, the ball, the boil on his finger. The half-term break in his therapy filled him with rage exploding out of him and leaving a hole in its wake. He tried to cover it, the ball at least and a tin on which he put it. He covered them with plasticine and called the result a 'monster'. But the covering was not complete. The dark blue ball showed through two holes in the plasticine. They looked at him, he said, with 'deathly eyes'.

Faced with the next gap in his treatment – the Christmas break – he again made a covering to stave off his rage. He asked Tustin for a large cardboard box: 'So that I can make a body', he explained, 'and dive right into it'. Later he said the box was a suit of armour to protect him from the 'monster with the hole'. Tustin gave him some more cardboard. He made it into a helmet and a gauntlet. As he did so he talked about his father, saying, 'Now, I'll take some of his hair', 'Now I'll take his ear', 'This is the nose'. It seemed he wanted to dive into his father, just as he had wanted to dive into Tustin. He got her to change seats with him. Then, when they changed back, he said, 'I expect I looked like you when I was sitting in your chair. Perhaps you are me and I am you'.

From his covering himself, as it were, to become Tustin or his father, and from his covering the ball with plasticine, Tustin speculated that his thus 'encapsulating' himself was a means of defending himself against his hole; he felt that the hole was made by the rage erupting out of him when he was faced with being separated from her during the half-term and Christmas breaks in his therapy.

Drawing on the theories of Bion and Bick, and on what she had learnt from her own and her previous patients' experience, Tustin contrasted his self-encapsulation with the baby who, taking in and feeling mothered inside, feels held together within his skin so he can begin to tolerate separation without fear of dissolution. If this fails, Tustin wrote, the child remains centred on outer bodily processes – as David was in being centred on, and preoccupied with the outward boil, pus and tits to the exclusion of what he might inwardly feel and think.

David's treatment ended in the early 1960s. Soon after, in September 1964, Arnold Tustin retired from Imperial College and was appointed to a post in Derby advising British Rail on problems they were having developing a high-speed rail service. He and Frances moved to nearby Ravenshead, and Frances worked a few miles away in a child guidance clinic in Nottingham. But Arnold suffered chronically from hay fever caused by the pollen of the silver birch trees in the area, and within a year they returned south – to Dorchester-on-Thames near Oxford and then to Tring. Here Frances resumed her private psychotherapy practice, worked in 1969–70 at a child guidance clinic in Aylesbury and supervised students on Mattie Harris's child psychotherapy course. One of them, recalling seeing Tustin for supervision in a flat in West Hampstead, described her as a 'rather small, round lady, dressed in purple, with a peaceful smiling face, who walked with a bit of a limp'.[14]

By the early 1970s Frances and Arnold had again moved house, to live in Great Missenden, Buckinghamshire, where in January 1975 she began treating another autistic boy, Peter. From him she learnt more about the importance of not colluding with the autistic child's encapsulating clinging to outer objects and shapes, and about ways in which such clinging stops inner feeling and thinking.

Inner thinking

Peter was the older of two children of an intelligent middle-class Jewish couple.[15] Tustin said that his mother was disappointed when he was born because he sucked so weakly at the breast he had to be bottle-fed. She was also depressed at her husband's work then taking him abroad for several months. When Peter was two their second child was born; six months later a psychotherapist, Anni Bergman, diagnosed Peter as one of the most severe cases of autism she had ever seen. He had no speech. He was extremely withdrawn. He had bizarre hand movements, walked on his toes and avoided looking at people. With the help of cognitive therapy he learnt to talk, but in a very restricted and stilted manner. And he learnt to hold a pencil. But by the time he started therapy with Tustin at the age of six he could neither draw nor write freely or spontaneously.

As his family lived far away in Oldham, Lancashire, Peter's sessions with Tustin in Great Missenden were restricted to weekends. He saw her in a consulting-room Arnold had made for her out of a stable in their garden. On first arriving in January 1975, Peter was carrying an enormous keyring with what looked like a hundred keys on it, all different sizes and shapes. He spent the next hour monotonously reciting nursery rhymes, stuffing toy animals into a shed and desultorily digging with a spade. He wanted to add the spade to his collection of things – to make Tustin and him the same. But Tustin did not agree to it. Refusing to collude and go along with him, she told him he could not take the spade with him. At this he panicked. He lay kicking on the floor with rage. Finally he went to the sand tray, picked up handfuls of sand and trickled it through his fingers, as though to take away the sensation on his hand.

At his fourth meeting with Tustin, on 1 February 1975, he drew round the keys. They were things he added to his body, she said, to plug the holes. He also added Tustin as a thing into whom he put questions to which he knew the answers and which he expected to pop out of her. He called her a vending machine. He thought of himself as a thing, as a toy crocodile. In one session he wrapped up the crocodile, encapsulating it. He put it into a plastic bag, laid it at the bottom of an empty goldfish bowl, then covered it with a piece of cardboard. On top of this he put a family of dolls and on top of them two plasticine figures. He called one 'God', the other a guard. Tustin likened the result to William Blake's engraving of *Behemoth and Leviathan*, one of the poet's illustrations for the Book of Job.

Blake's engraving shows God with two guardian angels at the top, a dragon at the bottom, and a huge beast with human ears in between where ordinary humanity mediates between body and soul or, as Tustin put it, between 'bestiality and hyperspirituality'. Two years into his therapy, this division emerged in Peter alternating between farting through his bottom and bubbling spit through his mouth. He talked of skunks sending out bad smells, and of his spit and whistling as a 'bubble of joy'. The stink and joy bubbles corresponded, Tustin wrote, to his goldfish bowl arrangement of God on top and a crocodile below. There seemed to be nothing – no mind – in between.

Shortly afterwards Peter spent a session using string to haul toy animals from one drawer of a chest of drawers to another higher up. She asked him if the drawers were like his body. He nodded. 'It looks as if the middle part is your tummy', she said. 'Oh no', he said deter-

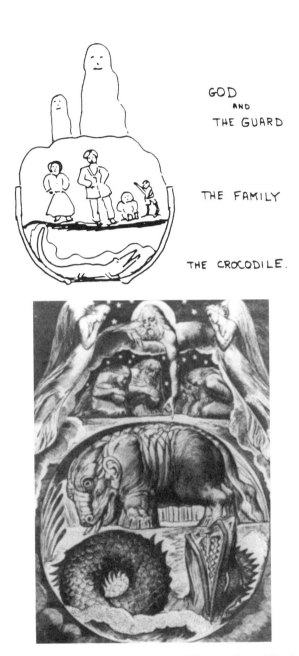

GOD
AND
THE GUARD

THE FAMILY

THE CROCODILE.

Peter's bowl and Blake's engraving of *Behemoth and Leviathan*

minedly, 'That part is missed out'. He went on hauling up the toy animals as Tustin, thinking aloud, talked to him about the missed-out part being the drawers Peter shared with the other children who came to see her. It was a part he did not know about, a part that was not him, she said. At this he again started moving the toys from the higher to the lower drawer. The toys were going round and round, she commented, without changing. Not a good way to grow up.

To this he said, 'It's changed inside my tummy'. Then, putting the toy animals on the string at the top, he moved his mouth as if eating. The toys were like food going in at the top and coming out of the bottom without his knowing what went on in between because he could not see or touch it. But that is where the changes take place, she said. 'They might get out', he replied, rubbing his belly-button. Perhaps he was frightened of what might get out of Tustin's tummy if it was unbuttoned. 'Monsters', he said.

At this Tustin talked with him about his fear of monsters in his own and his mother's tummy, and of food being changed inside into shit. 'Digested', he said. Tustin then told him how she watched and described his pulling up the toy animals. She turned it over in the tummy of her mind, digesting it. She shared with him what she did, just as he shared with her what he did. And from this shared middle thing, she said, something new came out. 'I suppose that's thinking', he said.

It was indeed. It marked his dawning recognition of himself and others having minds in which things outside could be taken in, thought about and digested, so he could change and grow and develop. His progress continued. He finished therapy, passed the 11+ and a difficult exam to a local private school. While at university he wrote to Tustin thanking her for releasing him from the 'prison of autism'.

Ordinarily occurring autism

Tustin included Peter's story in her book *Autistic States in Children* (1981). It was based on her previous years' teaching in England and South America and at Rome University's Institute of Child Neuropsychiatry, where her work was first best known.[16] Around 1976 she and Arnold moved from Great Missenden to a bungalow in Orchard Lane, Amersham.

Paying tribute to Bion, Tustin described – perhaps in part on the basis of what she had learnt from David's dead-making self-encapsulation and from Peter's resistance to thinking – how she too had once been 'half-dead', and of how Bion had brought her alive, and provoked her to think for herself. He impelled her to have a mind of her own,[17] and to stop mindlessly complying with others. As a child she had gone along with the submissiveness preached by her mother's religion:

> Make me Lord, obedient, mild
>   As becomes a little child
> All day long, in every way
> Teach me what to do and say.[18]

Now she wrote of how Bion had helped dissolve her encapsulating compliance. She compared the effect to the spiritual transformation undergone by Christian in John Bunyan's allegory *The Pilgrim's Progress*.

Soon after finishing her analysis with Bion, she had suffered a setback for which had had a brief analysis with Stanley Leigh.[19] It taught her, she said, about the roots of autism in herself, and led to her writing her first book on the subject, *Autism and Childhood Psychosis*, first published in 1972. It also led her in the 1980s to write about the ordinarily occurring roots of autism in mothers often becoming depressed following childbirth. She suggested that the greater frequency of autism in boys may be due to mothers experiencing the birth of a son as a more depressing loss than the birth of a daughter. She also illustrated how depression in mothers can lead to their babies withdrawing into quasi-autistic blankness. An example, she wrote, was a three-week-old baby who, faced with his depressed mother's utter lack of response to his liveliness, withdrew into what the observer described as 'helplessness, face averted, body curled-up and motionless'.[20]

In her article 'The growth of understanding', published in 1984, Tustin noted ways in which we all use 'autistic objects and shapes'. She described how babies and toddlers often use their piss, shit, spit and vomit, or the food in their mouths, to mediate between their subjective and objective, inner and outer worlds. Emphasizing the significance universally accorded the resulting shapes, she recounted the Scandinavian myth of Odin, who created the world by leaning over a bottomless chasm until the swirling mists formed into a shape below. We too know about such shapes, she said: feel your bottom pressing against the chair in which you are sitting – wriggle and the shape changes. It is personal to you, just as the toddler's shapes are personal to him. Again she cited mythology. She reminded her readers of a current television programme based on the Chinese myth *Monkey*, in which a monkey and a faceless creature called 'shape-changer' go into the belly of a monster, emerge and reunite with a man to contain, as Tustin put it, his otherwise ungrounded thinking and feeling. She talked of normally occurring shape-making predispositions as 'primary moulds' containing and constituting the precursor of 'me' sensations. She described how these moulds change – through drawing, music and so on – into perceptions of what is 'not-me'. Others have since likened the shapes she described to what the literary theorist and psychoanalyst Julia Kristeva calls the semiotic rhythms between mother and child that precede and form the living texture of symbolism and speech.[21]

In 1984, in recognition of her achievements in psychoanalysis, Tustin was elected to honorary affiliate membership of the British Psycho-Analytical Society. That year she began to break with the psychoanalytical theory of Margaret Mahler, which she had first learnt in Boston. Mahler called the baby's initial oneness with the mother 'primary autism'.[22] Tustin now rejected this term as too redolent of pathology. To emphasize the universality and normality of the baby's initial oneness with the mother she called it 'undifferentiated autosensuousness'[23] and described it as a 'continuous, rhythmical ebb and flow'.[24] Children recovering from autism would depict breaks in this flow as 'rushing water or explosive fluids and gases'.[25] She quoted Martin Luther describing his analogous break with his mother church as 'the darkness and the hole'.[26] She quoted Emily Brontë describing the agony of emerging from just such a hole:

> Oh dreadful is the check – intense the agony –
> When the ear begins to hear, and the eye begins to see;
> When the pulse begins to throb, the brain to think again;
> The soul to feel the flesh, the flesh to feel the chain.[27]

W. B. Yeats, she said, evoked similar agony in his poem 'The Second Coming', especially in the line, 'Things fall apart; the centre cannot hold'.[28] So too did Sylvia Plath, who described herself hugging the 'grudge, ugly and prickly, and sad sea-urchin' to shield herself from broken oneness with her mother following her brother's birth when she was two and a half.[29] Plath's husband, Ted Hughes, described the same brokenness, the spilling, the dissolution in his unpunctuated poem Wodwo:

> I seem
> separate from the ground and not rooted but dropped
> out of nothing casually I've no threads
> fastening me to anything[30]

To these literary examples Tustin added further examples from her patients. She quoted an anorexic patient likening her sense of being dropped to a 'waterfall falling and falling out of control into a bottomless abyss, into boundless space, into nothingness'.[31] Another anorexic took refuge in an image of herself as a rock:

> I have no need of friendship
> Friendship causes pain
> The laughter and its loving I disdain
> I am a rock, I am an island.[32]

Tustin thus sought to highlight autistic processes to which we are all prone. Therapists, she insisted, should be in touch with these processes in themselves so as to be alive to them in their patients.

Having long changed and developed her theories on the basis of what she had learnt from other therapists, her own experience and from the experience of her patients, Tustin now took her theory another step forward: contrary to what Mahler believed, she found that children do not usually experience themselves as one with their mothers, but have a rudimentary awareness of their separateness from their mothers from the very beginning of life. Klein, Tustin pointed out, had always maintained this.[33] The converse – initial oneness and lack of separation and difference – is the exception, not the rule. Emphasizing findings to this effect, Tustin also cited research characterizing failure to recognize difference – that others have minds of their own – as the effect of developmental delay in acquiring what researchers now called a 'theory of mind'.[34] She described the ingenious experiments devised to demonstrate that autistic children are less able to imagine others thinking differently from themselves than normal children or those with Down's syndrome.[35] She incorporated these findings into her book *The Protective Shell in Children and Adults* (1990).

Tustin continued teaching in England and abroad, but was too ill to attend a conference organized in France in 1993 in honour of her eightieth birthday. Throughout her life she had often been ill. Her husband's nephew Graham remembers that when they first met in 1948 she was hobbling on a stick. She suffered miscarriages, diabetes and polyomyalgia rheumatica, for which she was treated with steroids which in turn made her ill with acute hypertension. But it was Arnold who died first – in January 1994. He was ninety-four. The two of them 'had been like two trees', she said, 'grown together for so long that their roots were inextricably bound up with one another, and so when one died the other would wither away soon after'.[36] That is exactly what happened: in August 1994 she was diagnosed as having cancer of the colon. Ill also with secondaries, she moved from the bungalow in Amersham into a nearby retirement home, Rayner's.

Towards the end, perhaps recalling her childhood closeness with her religious mother, she talked of writing about sensation and spirituality for *Nature*.[37] But the article was never written. She died on 11 November 1994. On 11 February 1995 former patients, friends and colleagues, including fellow members of the Association of Child Psychotherapists and of the Squiggle Foundation (to whose journal *Winnicott Studies* she had often contributed), gathered in the Tavistock Clinic to celebrate her life and work. Her once autistic patient, Peter, was also there. Although somewhat odd and insensitive,[38] he was in good condition – a testimony to Tustin's achievement in using what she learnt from her own and her patients' experience, and from other Kleinian, post-Kleinian and non-Kleinian theorists about helping children and adults shed the inside-out armouring of autism. In doing so she quoted Hanna Segal, particularly her innovative theories regarding symbolism and psychosis.

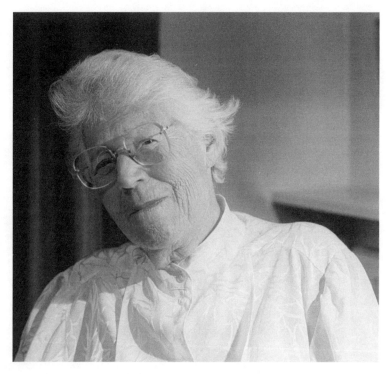

Hanna Segal, 1995/6

9 Hanna Segal: Symbolism and Psychosis

While Frances Tustin's insights into anorexia and autism arguably stemmed from her early closeness with her mother, Hanna Segal's theories about symbolism and psychosis may have started with her early ambition to follow her father in becoming a writer. Whatever the source of her theories, their major import is to show how facing separation, loss and inner reality enables us to generate and use the symbols needed to write and communicate successfully with others. Segal has used this observation to advance psychoanalytic treatment of psychosis, mania and depression. She has also used it to advance the applications of psychoanalysis to literature and politics.

From Poland to Proust[1]

Segal's father, Czeslaw Poznanski, wrote an important book about nineteenth-century French sculpture. He began it in 1905 after leaving Warsaw for Paris because of a strike of Polish students against the Russian authorities. On subsequently returning to Warsaw he gave up writing and became a lawyer like his father. He married Isabella Weintraub, and their first child, Wanda, was born in 1916. While he was on a political assignment in Łódź, their second child, Hanna (known as 'Hanka' by her friends and family), was born on 20 August 1918. Three months later the family returned to Warsaw, where Wanda died of scarlet fever when Hanna was two.

Happier childhood memories include the beauty of her mother, Isabella, and her lack of vanity, in contrast to the vanity of her mother's friend Mrs Sokolnicka, who was one of the first psychoanalysts in Paris and figured in André Gide's novel *The Counterfeiters*. Segal remembers as a child being fascinated by Mrs Sokolnicka having six black cats. She also remembers talking in her early teens with Mrs Sokolnicka about psychoanalysis.

By then she had started school – when she was ten – and reluctantly moved to Geneva two years later, when her father gave up his law practice to take up a post as editor on the *Journal des nations*. All the moves of her life have been forced on her, she says; nevertheless she enjoyed swimming in the lake there. (Indeed, now in her eighties, she still likes swimming.) She also enjoyed learning more about European culture at the progressive international school she attended in Geneva. But she wanted to return to Poland. Appealing to her father's Polish patriotism, she persuaded him to allow her to return to Warsaw to complete her last two years of secondary school, where she studied French philosophy, particularly that of Pascal, for her diploma thesis. She later supplemented these studies with reading German philosophy and all Freud's writings available in French or Polish translation. Discovering psychoanalysis, she says, was a 'godsend'. It combined her three major interests – literature, science and politics. This last – specifically outrage at widespread poverty in Poland – led her to join the student section of the Polish Socialist Party when she was seventeen, even though this was illegal because she was still at school.

For further education Hanna initially thought of studying art or literature. But then these seemed too academic and abstract. Sociology and psychology were more appealing as a means of doing something socially useful. She thought of working in prison administration, but her father advised her against becoming dependent on a salary. 'If you want to reform something', he told her, 'find yourself a profession which makes you completely independent'.[2] She opted for medicine, not writing, she explains, because 'I recognised that you could only produce something of lasting worth in literature if you had an extraordinary gift, whereas I realised that even with modest ability, without having to be first class, as a doctor you can do a reasonable amount of good just by doing your job'.[3] So in 1936 she started studying medicine. In her second year at Warsaw University she met Bychowsky, a lecturer in neurology and one of Poland's very few psychoanalysts at that time. He told her that to train as an analyst she should go to Vienna. But she did not want to go there. Instead she continued studying in Warsaw. Meanwhile political factors, including the growth of fascism in Poland, and the avowed fascism of the Swiss President, who was determined to destroy the *Journal des nations*, led to Hanna's father being expelled from Switzerland. He and Hanna's mother moved to Paris, where they were living, hard up and stateless, when Hanna visited them in the summer of 1939. The outbreak of war prevented her from returning to Warsaw. So she stayed in Paris and continued her studies at the École de Médecine. Here she established contact with a cousin, Paul Segal. As children they had disliked each other; now he was studying physics and they became friends.

But again she had to move. The German occupation of France in July 1940 forced her and her parents to move to London, where they settled in a flat in Earl's Court. At first it seemed likely she would have to repeat her second MB at Manchester University. But, with the opening of a Polish Medical School at Edinburgh University, she was able to go straight into her fourth year of medical training there. While in Edinburgh, she met W. R. D. Fairbairn. He told her about the Controversial Discussions then going on in the British Psycho-Analytical Society. He also gave her Klein's and Anna Freud's books about child analysis, which decided Hanna to train as a Kleinian. Fairbairn helped her with this by introducing her to David Matthew, a doctor in Edinburgh who had been analysed by Klein and agreed to take her on for a nominal fee. She stayed in analysis with him until she completed her medical training a year later, moved to London, and took a job in Paddington Children's Hospital. Determined to be analysed by Klein, she applied. Klein accepted her despite the fact that at first she was unable to pay the £20 a month fee. This was remedied six months later, when Hanna got a job with the Ministry of Health at Long Grove in Epsom (where, under the auspices of the Polish Government in Exile, she and her boss, Dr George Bram, organized a mental rehabilitation centre for its Polish soldier inmates).

In 1941 Hanna also began training at the London Institute of Psycho-Analysis, where she was supervised by Paula Heimann and Joan Riviere. Having qualified as a psychoanalyst in 1945, she immediately began training in child analysis, with supervision from Klein and Bick. Earlier that spring, her mother died at the age of fifty-four; Hanna continued to live with her father in Earl's Court. Soon they were joined by Paul Segal who had become a mathematician. On 16 November 1946 Paul and Hanna married and settled in Queen's Gate.

The next year, pregnant with their first child, Daniel (born on 26 October 1947, and now a mathematician at All Souls, Oxford), Segal presented her first paper to the British Psycho-Analytical Society. It was about the subject which had first led her to become a psychoanalyst, namely her preoccupation with what makes for great literature, and her lack of confidence in becoming great in this field herself. Freud, she noted, had never said what makes literature or art great or good. Drawing on Klein's theory of the depressive position, she filled in this lacuna in Freudian theory. She argued that great art or literature is constituted through recognition of love and of hateful destruction of loved figures within, impelling artists and writers to restore and repair these figures in what they create.

This has perhaps never been better expressed, Segal maintained, than by Proust in *Remembrance of Things Past*. At the end of its concluding volume, *Time Regained*, the narrator faces the ageing and dying of all those he has known and loved. In doing so he tells the reader of the impulse that inspired his novel – his repeated confrontation with oblivion of the past by the present and future inspiring him to generate the personal images and symbols needed to transform what is factually dead and gone into the living world of his novel. Or, as Proust's narrator puts it: 'I had to recapture from the shade that which I had felt, to reconvert it into its psychic equivalent. But the way to do it, the only one I could see, what was it – but to create a work of art?'[4]

Quoting Proust, Segal argued that creativity is inhibited to the extent that the writer or artist is unable to face the 'shade' of separation, death and loss. She illustrated the point with clinical examples. They included a woman writer who suffered from both anorexia and a writing block that was not relieved, Segal says, until the writer faced her inner loss as she did in associations to a dream: 'A baby has died or grown up – she didn't know which – and as a result her breasts were full of milk. She was feeding a baby of another woman, whose breasts were dry'.[5] Her associations included facing the loss of being weaned from, and losing, Segal with the end of her analysis. With this she felt more confident about writing, 'provided', she said, 'I can go on being sad for a while, without being sick and hating food'.[6]

Writing and art depend not only on being able to face sadness and inner loss, Segal added. They also depend on writers and artists communicating to others their experience of inner emptiness, fear and destruction. Quoting Rainer Maria Rilke, she insisted, 'Beauty is nothing but the beginning of terror that we are still just able to bear'.[7] She ended the talk with the topic of sculpture, citing Rodin's claim that art entails facing and transforming ugliness into beauty, just as, Segal noted, Freud claimed Michelangelo's achievement in his sculpture of Moses lay in his both facing and transforming wrath.

Segal is above all a psychoanalyst. And it was with a psychoanalytic case history that she launched her next breakthrough in advancing psychoanalytic understanding of symbolism, in her paper for membership of the British Psycho-Analytical Society, given in 1949 and published the following year. Her second child, Michael, was born the next year on 31 July 1950.

Symbolic equations

In her membership paper Segal provided the first case history that used Klein's ideas to treat a schizophrenic successfully and the first statement of what has come to be known as her theory of symbolic equations. Schizophrenia, or psychosis, she said, involves equating symbols with the objects they symbolize. To illustrate the point she described a patient, Edward. Before coming into analysis he had gone to a public school and won a scholarship to university which he was unable to take up because of the war. When he was eighteen he was called up and sent to India. But officer training in the Engineers proved too much for him. Failing to get a commission, and derided as a fool by one of the officers, he resigned to become a private. But this also proved too much. He broke down, heard voices, complained his eyes had stopped working and wrote a letter to the Colonel denouncing a biologist who, he said, was determined to destroy the world. He was hospitalized and returned to England where he was diagnosed as suffering from rapidly deteriorating schizophrenia.

After a few days in a military hospital Edward was taken by his parents to be treated in a private nursing home. It was here, in the early 1940s, that Segal began analysis with him, five times a week. The only thing he spontaneously asked at their first meeting was whether London was all right because India had been completely changed. Segal replied by explaining that he felt he had changed and that the world was changing with him. 'Yes', he said, 'I have been changed'. Twenty years old, he treated inner and outer reality as though they were the same. His failure to differentiate between them was a major feature of the first, acute stage of his illness.

Initially Segal evidently meant no more to him internally than the external furniture in the room where they met. How cut off and mis-understood he must feel, Segal said, to which he replied that all the prisoners felt that way. Prisoners in Germany sent him voices, he added. Being a prisoner was no different from seeming to be one. His conflation of seeming and being was also evident in his one day bringing to his meeting with Segal a canvas stool that he had made in occupational therapy. Embarrassed, as though the stool were no different from a stool of shit, he blushed and stammered. He was like another patient, Segal said, who, when he was asked why he no longer played the violin, retorted, 'Fancy masturbating in public',[8] as though the violin and his penis were the same.

As for Edward, not only did he equate symbols with what they symbolized but he was also fearful of change. He longed to keep Segal good, loved and unchanging. But he also dreaded loving her lest dependence on her make him hate her; if they became too close, he might infect her with his madness. Talking about these feelings and his sense of isolation, however, he began to get better, and after three months of analysis was able to go home.

But he then felt intense rage and despair at finding that, far from having left his delusions and hallucinations behind in the hospital, they were still with him. Whereas Segal's US counterparts evaded confronting such negative feelings in their schizophrenic patients, Segal confronted them directly. She talked to Edward about his fear that she was just as much of an enemy as he felt the other doctors had been in the hospital. She also talked to him about his longing for her to prove herself his ally and friend.

Talking through these feelings, Edward soon recovered sufficiently to see Segal in her consulting-room in Queen's Gate. Again, however, he was initially fearful at yet another change in his treatment setting. He walked anxiously around the room, said that a little bottle on her table contained poison, and that the little ivory skulls she had on her mantelpiece might be the skulls of patients she had killed. But then he added that he knew this was not true.

This was the first time, in Segal's hearing, that he distinguished his inner delusions from outer reality. A few days later he was able to use the couch. But he remained physically tense and rigid with anxiety. He was able to free associate, however, and soon his treatment became like that of a neurotic – a matter of interpreting his inner phantasies and defences. And, within a year of the start of his treatment, his equation of external reality with the internal reality of his delusions ceased. All that remained of his delusions was an encapsulated 'buzz', as he put it, split off from his growing awareness of good and bad not as things but as feelings, images and memories within him.

Edward spent four years in analysis, ending it partly because of family pressure to take up his long ago offered place at university. Having attended an extramural course, he got a degree, married, had a family and an adventurous – although not entirely successful – career. He remained well for many years, but in 1968 suffered another schizophrenic breakdown caused by external pressure. Remembering and retaining within him sufficient good feelings for Segal, he sought her help. As she did not have a vacancy he saw one of her colleagues, with whom he did well.

Meanwhile Segal had followed up his wartime analysis with other clinical work bearing on the relation between inner and outer reality.

This included writing about the inner impact on one of her neurotic patients of her moving her consulting-room in early 1948 (the family left Queen's Gate for Clifton Hill in St John's Wood, where Klein was also living). Segal's patient wanted to deny the move. He wanted to control everything and keep it static. Having told her in a previous session about a phantasy of making love to the dead, he now dreamt that Segal was a static wooden doll to whom he wanted to make love. But making Segal dead and unchanging threatened to do the same to him: he dreamt not only that she was a wooden doll but that, in making love to her, his penis became wooden too.[9]

In 1954 Segal was appointed as a training analyst. In her next paper, 'Depression in the schizophrenic', published in 1956, she described a patient, whom I will call Sarah, who had suffered hallucinations since she was at least four. Her father committed suicide when she was fifteen and a year later she started analysis, suffering from what Segal called 'hebephrenia'. To highlight the conflation of inner and outer reality Segal described a session with Sarah, two years into her analysis. It began with Sarah seemingly hallucinating that she was her father, as both God and the devil. She then picked up imaginary things from the carpet, dancing around the room as she did so. Segal compared her to Shakespeare's Ophelia who, the more she dances and intertwines the flowers she picks, the sadder she makes everyone around her. Telling Sarah that she, like Ophelia, externalized her unbearable inner sadness into others, Sarah replied that what was so unbearable in Ophelia was the intertwining of her sanity and madness. 'She was irresponsible, like a child', she said, 'she did not know the difference'.[10]

Generalizing from Sarah's case, and from that of Edward, Segal went on to formalize her theory of symbolic equations in what is her best-known and most important essay, published in 1957.[11] In it she developed Klein's theory of symbolism. Writing about her four-year-old 'schizophrenic' patient Dick (see pp. 18–19 above), Klein argued that symbolization of others – in the first place symbolization of the mother – is impelled by concern to preserve them from hatred and attack. But if anxiety is too great, as occurred with Dick, this process fails to get going. It becomes paralysed and stuck.

To this observation Segal added that symbolization may develop but become disturbed in psychosis by the patient projecting himself or herself into, and identifying with other people and things, including equating them with what they symbolize. Edward had equated the canvas stool he made in occupational therapy with the faeces the stool symbolized for him. Sarah, when she was ill, symbolized her earlier phantasies of herself and her mother devouring each other or her father in a story she herself told as a child about Lancashire witches. Later, however, overcome by anxiety, she imagined the witches were real. She projected them into Segal and identified with them in her. She assumed Segal knew about them without her having to tell her. She even thought Segal was one of the witches. She equated the witches and the people they symbolized – herself, her mother and Segal.

Facing death

In 1958 the Segals had to move again, as the lease on their St John's Wood home had expired; they moved to 3 Lyndhurst Road, Hampstead. That year Segal published an essay in which she poignantly described a patient facing the ultimate move – from life to death. This essay centred on an elderly man from Rhodesia who, confronted with the increasing likelihood of his dying when he reached the age of seventy, suffered a psychotic breakdown. Psychiatric treatment left him depressed and hypochondriacal. It also left him subject to paranoid delusions and to outbursts of insane rage. His son, who was studying in London and was concerned about him, arranged for him to have analysis and he began treatment with Segal nearly two years after he had first broken down.

By then he was seventy-three. Analysis revealed that his breakdown had been triggered by his first visit to his son in London, when he re-established contact with one of his younger brothers. He had left his poverty-stricken orthodox Jewish family in the Ukraine when he emigrated to Rhodesia, and now learnt that they had perished in Hitler's concentration camps. His breakdown was also triggered by his discovery, on returning from London to Rhodesia, that a man he had bribed for several years to secure business deals for him had been taken into custody for dishonesty. Terrified that he too might be caught, he became convinced that the newspapers and radio were reporting him and that people in the street were laughing at him. Most of all, it transpired, he had broken down because his ageing and approaching death had overwhelmed his previous defences against facing hatred and loss. These defences included denial, splitting and idealization, all of which became evident in his analysis.

As a child, it turned out, he had idealized his father and brother by splitting off all his negative feelings about them into his mother and into his other siblings. As an adult he idealized his son. Now, as a patient, he idealized Segal. He split off his negative feelings about her into Rhodesia. He also split them off into his son-in-law, who, he complained, had sent him to England to die of the cold. Following the first holiday break in his analysis, however, he was less often dominated by dividing good and bad. He began locating both in Segal. He experienced her as the source of both warmth and life, coldness and death. 'Doctor', he said one day, 'when you look at me with your kind eyes I can feel you drawing the illness out of me and throwing it out of the window'. But he also complained at the very next session: 'You can't imagine how it [Segal and his illness] got into me, how it squeezed me, how it burned me'.[12]

Gradually, however, he came to experience these contrary feelings alongside each other in him. Knowing about his own inner goodness and badness, and his own love and hate, culminated in his shaking his fist and angrily shouting in one of his sessions about his long dead parents: 'How did they dare to have a new baby [when he was two] when they could not feed the ones they had!'[13] With this a tremor, which looked Parkinsonian and had bothered him for several years, ceased. He became outwardly more calm. He was also more able to face his previously numbed inner feelings of guilt, loss and depression. This included tracing with Segal how, in 1939, he had secretly begun drinking to numb himself against his guilt at not having brought his family out of the Ukraine with him to Rhodesia; and his fear, following his business colleague's recent exposure, that he too would be exposed, in his case for having left his family to perish.

He became able to experience his actual rather than imagined guilt. No longer numbing himself with drink or with phantasies of being caught, he experienced the all too real guilt of having as a child reviled his mother as cold and rejecting, as an excuse for turning away from her and idealizing his father. Awareness of his guilt led him to become aware of his positive as well as negative feelings for his mother, of his appreciation for all the hard work she had put into keeping the family going through the poverty they suffered when he was a boy. He mourned her loss. He also mourned the life he too would soon lose. More immediately he anticipated mourning losing Segal when his analysis ended after eighteen months. In a session during his last week with her, he represented the good and bad that he now faced as together in him: he saw himself as a jug that was old and unprepossessing but also contained goodness – beer or milk.

In a postscript she later added to his case, Segal described how he returned to Rhodesia and remained in excellent health for the next eleven years. The evening before he died he told his wife that he at last inwardly believed (as opposed to simply knowing as an external fact) that their son was indeed in London. Now really and truly believing and knowing about his separation from, and loss of his son, and the emptiness it left within him, he fell asleep. In the middle of the night he woke up saying he was hungry. After eating a sandwich and drinking some milk his wife brought him, he again went to sleep, this time for ever.

Manic and megalomaniac denial

On 24 November 1960 Segal gave birth to her third and last child, Gabriel (who now teaches philosophy at King's College, London). She went on to give lectures to third-year students at London's Institute of Psycho-Analysis. They formed the basis of her first book, *Introduction to the Work of Melanie Klein*. In it she illustrated how, rather than face death and loss as her Rhodesian patient came to do, we may evade them through manic excitement and denial.

Manic denial, she said, involves turning away from recognizing dependence on others. It involves turning away from divided feelings of love and hate, and from inner reality generally, by instead culti-vating outer control, triumph and contempt. As an example she cited a patient who, early in his analysis, laughingly recounted a dream about a man in a barber's shop being shaved by a monkey. The man, he said, had a little kitten at home who could shave him much better. He was called Joe, just like the man who looked after the patient when he was a child, and whom he later failed to visit when he became old and ill. The kitten reminded him of his girlfriend, Kitty. He felt she was much better than Segal who, in his dream, he man-ically dismissed and triumphed over as a contemptible and laughable monkey barber.[14]

In an essay published in 1972 Segal related another example of a man manically denying inner loss through outward contempt. She described him as controlling and 'niggly'. On one occasion he began a session grumbling about the tobacco smoke in her consulting-room, the colour of her dress and the untidy way she let her maid run up the stairs when he came in. He went on to say that he and his wife had decided not to go away that summer, as they had suf-fered so many petty annoyances on holiday the previous year. He then told Segal a dream in which he, his wife, and their child were bothered by wasps in a lovely field of buttercups. Their yellow colour, he said, reminded him of a field of daffodils to which his uncle had taken him and some other children when he was four. They had gath-ered the flowers in armfuls. But on the way home they became bored, tore the flowers apart, threw them at each other and then threw them out of the window, littering the street where he lived. In Segal's view, his memory of triumphantly and contemptuously tearing up the flowers was a manic response to anticipating losing her over the holiday break. Its defensive character was rendered particularly vivid to Segal through her experience of a three-year-old in analysis, who similarly responded to a holiday break by tearing things up – not flowers but paper.[15]

Far more extreme than these examples, however, was the megalomaniac defence of another patient, George. He came into analysis with Segal when he was forty-four. He felt a mission to train as a priest, for which he believed he had been specially chosen by God, and he was afraid that his obsessional rituals, chronic indecision and doubt might stop him achieving the efficiency needed for him to enter a seminary. Born in 1917, he had been suddenly weaned when he was six weeks old because his mother did not want breastfeeding him to get in the way when his soldier father came home briefly from the war. Before his return she wrote saying, 'George cried for the breast but I didn't give it to him'.[16] Soon after going back to the front his father was killed. Almost immediately after that, she too was lost to George. She went abroad for a year, possibly to nurse in France. George's earliest memories, however, were not of losing his mother and father but of imagining himself to be the Pope, or President of the World. He could remember feeling bereft only once – on first going to boarding school when he was eight. But what he most remembered from prep school was it being the time he first became aware of his greatness – his genius for strategy. In analysis with Segal, this included a scheme, which he called 'operation anti-homosexuality': he planned to pick up all London's potentially attractive men so as to get them 'off his chest'.

It was only during the fifth year of his analysis that his belief in his genius began to disintegrate. He dreamt that a mountain of sand started crumbling under him. He dreamt that a big black dog, whom he referred to as 'delusional George', was chasing and determined to kill a tiny dog, 'baby Georgie'. He himself, he said, had nearly been killed. Two days before a brief interruption in his analysis he had gone to see his favourite lesbian prostitute, Jackie. He had played Dutch uncle to Jackie and her friend Betty, drunk a bottle of whisky, and talked to the two women about love and hate. But then he became completely impotent. Jackie had stroked him and said, 'Why don't you lie on your side, dear, you seemed to be doing better that way'. Her kindness and motherliness enraged him. He rushed away, intending to smash a bottle through Segal's window, but then rushed off to Piccadilly. There he picked up a man to whom he also talked about love and hate. He told him that he, George, was the murderer in a recently much publicized case involving a prostitute killed in the town where George had studied theology. An argument ensued about money in which George's pick-up became completely furious, and crazily danced around the room shouting, 'You are the murderer of all these women! I am going to kill you!' Hearing the noise, the land-lord of the hotel where they were staying intervened, whereupon George left.

From these and other incidents and dreams it gradually emerged that George's megalomaniac belief in being a genius strategist was the means by which he sought to stave off the crying and rage he had felt as a tiny baby on being weaned, and the terror that his crying and rage had been the cause of his then almost immediately losing his father and mother. According to Segal, it was to fend off the death and destruction seemingly done by his enraged and crying 'baby Georgie' self, that he generated his larger-than-life, 'delusional George' self. This figure was so self-sufficient and grand it cut him off from his mother when she eventually returned; he was not quite two at the time. It also cut him off from others when he was grown up because he feared that they might retaliate against him for having made them – his pick-up, for instance – the outer repository of his inner murderous crying and rage, from which he had first cut himself off as a baby.

Becoming aware in analysis of the delusional nature of his grandiose self was also terrifying. He dreamt that he was in an enor-mous completely empty room. All his genius amounted to was fifty years of empty nothingness. His 'delusional George' self had com-pletely stopped his 'baby Georgie' self from developing, achieving or creating anything real inside or out. Gradually, however, he became more able to experience Segal, as he had experienced the landlord in the pick-up incident, as an outsider containing the rage and murderousness he could not bear to know about within himself. This included experiencing Segal containing the hatred she felt for him on his coldly announcing, 'Hitler knew how to deal with you people'.[17] Gradually it became possible for him to take in her con-taining his outwardly projected hatred and rage, against which he had defended himself with his delusions of being a genius. As a result the danger of these feelings exploding into suicide or murder con-siderably decreased.

Literature, politics and art

What, meanwhile, had become of Segal's own early ambitions? True to her early involvement in literature, politics and art, she has often applied her clinical insights into all three subjects. In 1974 she pub-lished an essay about the manic control, triumph, contempt and

denial of inner reality depicted by William Golding in *The Spire*.[18]
The novel centres on Jocelin, the dean of a cathedral, driven by
megalomaniac belief that he has been especially appointed by God
to have a 400-foot spire built onto his cathedral. Ruthlessly he drives
the master builder, who is called Mason, to build it. Triumphing over
him and everyone else with his belief that he has an angel on his side,
Jocelin contemptuously derides not only Mason and his wife Rachel,
but Pangall and his wife Goody, for their childlessness. Jocelin denies
inner psychic reality. He ignores Goody's grief at the loss of Pangall
when he disappears and dies in a pit on the building site. He denies
the depression and alcoholism to which Mason succumbed as the
possibility of the spire crashing down and destroying everything
became increasingly likely. He denies and ignores the stink of rotting
corpses caused by the building work opening up the ground and
tombs below the cathedral. He denies the lack of any foundation,
apart from shifting mud, that the building work reveals.

As it proceeds the spire bends and leans so perilously that building has to stop. It will never be made. Jocelin's creative ambition
comes to nothing. He discovers that his belief in having been especially appointed by God to have the tower built, and to become dean
of the cathedral, is an illusion. He learns his deanship was secured
for him by his aunt as a gift from her lover, the king, in celebration
of their love-making. It was not his own divinely inspired doing. He
despairs. Facing inner collapse, he tells Mason: 'I'm a building with
a vast cellarage where the rats live; and there's some kind of blight
on my hands. I injure everyone I touch, particularly those I love'.[19]
But it is too late. His project is a failure. It cannot be revived. By
contrast, Segal considered Golding's novel a success because, unlike
Jocelin's spire, it grows out of facing and symbolizing an inner world
– represented by the world of the cathedral and its people – of love
and destruction, grief and death.

In 1977–8 Segal was the third Freud Memorial Visiting Professor
of Psychoanalysis at UCL. In her inaugural lecture, 'Psychoanalysis
and freedom of thought', she spoke of widespread resistance (like
that of Jocelin in Golding's novel) in politics, science and culture
generally – as well as in psychoanalysis – to facing what is going on,
inside and out.[20]

In subsequent essays Segal further illustrated this theme with the
example of Joseph Conrad. Before becoming an established writer,
he was depressed by his failure to find a post as a ship's captain,
although qualified for the position. In 1889 he at last achieved a captaincy – of the *Otago* in Bangkok. It was then that he began writing.
But he soon became bored and after a year gave up the job because
it was preventing him from fulfilling a long-standing ambition to

go to Africa. While waiting for a suitable post to take him there, he visited his uncle and guardian, Thaddeus Brobowski, and spent his time writing feverishly. By the time he got the post he wanted, commanding a small ship going up the Congo, he had written six chapters of his first novel, *Almayer's Folly*. But he was racked by depression and illness on the journey, cut short his contract and returned to Europe, ill and shattered. In 1891 his depression lifted slightly on his taking up a position as first mate on the *Torrens*. But he then had to take up the humiliating position of second mate on another boat so as to be able to visit his uncle, who was now dying. It was only following his death, in 1894, that Conrad at last completed *Almayer's Folly* and arranged for it to be published the following year.

These are the outward facts. His increasingly facing their inward effect is conveyed in three novellas, beginning with *The Heart of Darkness* (1902). In it, said Segal, Conrad depicted his aborted facing of his inner world in the person of the narrator, Marlowe, who voyages into the interior of the Congo and retreats from the hellish savagery, cannibalism and corruption he finds there, as does the grandiose Mr Kurtz. Kurtz dies protesting 'The horror, the horror', never having realized his much talked of promise as an artist, writer or musician.

Conrad further confronted his inner world in *The Secret Sharer* (1912), which tells the story of a ship's captain who is much more persistent than Marlowe and Kurtz in facing his inner world's negative aspects. They are represented, said Segal, by the captain's double, a drowning man, whom he rescues, takes on board, and discovers to be a murderer. Dreading that others might discover his counterpart's existence, he keeps his presence secret but then becomes almost crazy with paranoid isolation from his crew, whose lives – together with his own – he risks by sailing close to the rocks of an island, Koh-ring, so as to get rid of his double by enabling him to jump overboard and swim ashore.

Segal considered that only with *The Shadow Line* (1917), did Conrad describe a character successfully persisting in facing his inner world. Subtitled *A Confession*, the novella begins with the narrator arriving in Bangkok, suffering from the 'green-sickness of late youth'.[21] Destroyed by envy and contempt – including contempt for a Captain Giles who helps the narrator get his first command – everything seems futile and pointless. But when he takes up the post *tedium vitae* soon gives way to manic excitement, almost immediately succeeded by disillusionment.

The crew and first mate, Burns, fall sick. Because of the narrator's triumph in getting the captaincy instead of him, Burns refuses to stay ashore, despite being desperately sick. As the voyage proceeds, he becomes increasingly ill and deluded. He is convinced that the previous captain (who the narrator learns led a life of unrestrained dissolution ending in insanity and death) has returned as an evil spirit to destroy everyone on board. Burns is convinced that battle must above all be done with the dead captain's ghost at latitude 8°20', the shadow line where his body was buried at sea. Worse still, the narrator discovers that before his predecessor died he emptied the ship's medicine bottles of quinine, sold it and replaced it with sand.

Facing the depths of despair, he begins to keep a diary. Recognizing his responsibility, he admits to the crew that he should have checked the ship's medical supplies before leaving shore. Facing his failure with them, the crew help him. His mate, Burns, battles successfully with the ghost of the dead captain. The ship passes the fatal latitude, and when they at last arrive in Singapore the narrator is a changed man. Now at last he can appreciate and feel grateful to Captain Giles for securing him his first command. Better still he brings ashore alive and well his once vengeful, triumphed-over and crazy but now convalescent *alter ego* – Burns. His achievement in facing and reconciling himself with his inner shortcomings is also mirrored in another figure – the ship's cook, Ransome – who, from the beginning, has known and faced the fact that he has a weak heart and may well die soon.

Segal not only used Conrad's writing to illustrate how creative communication can come from facing good and bad, life and death, within us, she also drew attention to its converse – the destruction, global as well as individual, resulting from failing to face what is going on, inside or out. In 1983, with the psychoanalyst Moses Laufer, she founded the British Association of Psychoanalysts for the Prevention of Nuclear War. Inaugurating its international counterpart in 1985, she spoke of our pervasive failure to face inner grief and the outer potential for global destruction made possible by the world's escalating arms race. Instead, she said, we tend to blur fantasy and reality, all the more so since grandiose inner illusions of total destruction can all too readily be realized outwardly through nuclear annihilation. We also tend to ignore and get rid of inner destruction by externalizing it into others. We make outsiders into ever more terrifying enemies in whose name we justify the arms race. We fuel it with fantasies of terror and deterrence. Knowing about inner reality, she urged, analysts must speak out. Not to do so would be a crime.[22]

Segal's next book, *Dream, Phantasy and Art* (1991), is devoted to aesthetics. Quoting Proust's assertion that 'a book is a vast graveyard where on most of the tombstones one can read no more the faded names',[23] she again described the inner love and loss that she has all along maintained must be faced for outward creativity to succeed. She illustrated the point with the example of Picasso, overcome with depression when he was nineteen on first seeing Velásquez's paintings, many years later fragmenting *Las meninas* and re-creating it in his own terms, just as he faced and symbolically re-created the destruction wrought by the Spanish Civil War in *Guernica*. The book also cites the experience of the biographer Richard Holmes. Holmes describes how he is initially impelled in his work by identifying with and idealizing his biographical subjects, as he did when he was eighteen in going on the same travels in the Cévennes as one of his first subjects, Robert Louis Stevenson. But identification is not enough. Doing the necessary research and writing depends, notes Holmes, on facing the loss involved in not being the same person as the subject he writes about. Segal ends *Dream, Phantasy and Art* with further examples from the visual arts. She describes patients stymied in their outer creativity by not facing their inner world. She contrasts one such patient with Hogarth, who, she writes, faced with deeply etched humour and sexuality the degradation and horror he depicts in his lithographs.

In 1991 the Gulf War impelled Segal again to write about politics.[24] The ending of the Cold War, she wrote, could have led us to stop externalizing – into the Soviet Union, for example – the destruction in England involved in its economic decline and widespread unemployment. Instead the government preferred to find a new outsider to demonize – Saddam Hussein. After the Gulf War, and not wanting to face the destruction in which it resulted, we are likely, she warned, to seek other outsiders in whose name to continue waging war and destruction.[25]

Segal went on to combine her lifelong involvement in politics and creativity in a talk to a conference in November 1992, in which she spoke about *Haroun and the Sea of Stories* (1990),[26] Salman Rushdie's first novel to follow the Iranian fatwah declared against him. In it Rushdie tells the story of Rashid who, in becoming renowned for his effervescent story-telling, fails to take heed of the misery around him, including that of his wife. She leaves him for their neighbour, a man who hates stories and story-tellers, just as the Ayatollah must have seemed to Rushdie to hate him. Blaming his father for his mother leaving them, Rashid's son, Haroun, complains that his stories are not even true. This silences Rashid. All he can say is 'Ark, ark, ark'. He does not regain his story-telling ability until Haroun – his son and counterpart – has crossed a twilight strip (analogous to Conrad's shadow line), has been imprisoned in a dark ship and then confronts the terrible feeling of hopelessness he discovers on first diving into a sea of stories.

Rushdie's novel is, essentially, a fable for children. Segal gave her talk about it in the same year that her fifth grandchild, Amber, was born. She was the first girl born into Hanna's and Paul's branch of the Segal family for a hundred years! Also in 1992, Hanna received the accolade of the Sigourney award for her outstanding contribution to psychoanalysis.

Symbolism revisited

Segal's outstanding contribution, as I have sought to explain, includes most significantly her pioneering account – particularly in her essays of 1947 and 1957 – of ways we variously face, and fail to face, loss and depression in our inner world in generating and using the symbols needed to communicate what is going on inwardly to others outside. Her work on symbolism did not stop with these essays. In August 1977, in a paper to the first psychoanalytic congress to be held in Israel, she returned to the theme of her essay of 1957.[27]

In that essay, as discussed above, she argued that in psychosis patients may projectively identify with people and things, and equate the latter with what they symbolize. In 'On symbolism' she supplemented her earlier theory with Bion's observations regarding mothers taking in, containing and digesting what their babies projectively put into them by way of love, hatred and knowledge. Bion argued that, if the baby is too full of hatred and envy of what is good and loved in the mother, he will be impeded from experiencing her as taking in and containing what is in him, so that he can take it back into himself as contained and containable by her (see p. 127 above). To this Segal added in her book *Klein* (1979) that the mother may so need to think of herself as perfect that she stops her baby's negative feelings getting into her. She may bolster her self-worth by treating her baby as worthless compared with her. She may thereby contribute and add to his envy of her, and to his difficulty in experiencing her as containing his feelings and making it bearable to know about them within himself.

In an essay of 1994 Segal summarized the development in the 1970s of her earlier theories about symbolization.[28] Entitled 'Phantasy and reality', it reminds her readers of Freud's theory that the baby first bridges the gap between his inner hunger and the outer absence of his mother by hallucinating – or dreaming – that she is there. Segal now added that in psychosis the gap between dreams and reality can become abolished by patients imagining that outer reality is one and the same as their inner hallucinations and phantasies about it. She cited the example of a patient, Mr B, who suffered from gastric ulcer. For as long as he could remember, he had also suffered a recurring nightmare of being attacked by elongated animals with crocodile mouths. They turned out to be an effect of his externalizing into them his inner image of himself screaming with colic as a baby when he was tightly swaddled into an elongated crocodile-like shape. Unable to contain his hate-filled screaming, he spewed it out into these crocodile-mouthed figures in his nightmare, and into an image of his wife's vagina as full of biting teeth.

Much happier is another example – that of a Mr C, who first came into analysis fearful of becoming schizophrenic. As his treatment progressed he experienced Segal taking in and containing what he said. Initially he felt she so much took in what he said that he did not have to remember it. Later, having experienced her containing his words and feelings, he felt more able to take them back into himself as contained and remembered by her. He felt more able to face what was going on within him. He symbolized the pleasure and pain of his resulting recognition of his difference and separation from her in a dream, in which, he told her:

> You were in Scotland and I was thrilled to see you. It was marvellous having you there. But it was not like the last occasion you were in Scotland. I had nothing to do with it. I did not even know what your lecture was to be about. It was a strange experience because I was so pleased to see you, and yet I felt so excluded. It was so awful not even knowing what you planned or what was on your mind.[29]

Segal concluded Mr C's story by reiterating her revised theory of symbolism. Again she argued that symbolism depends on experiencing the mother taking in and containing what we put into her – just as Mr C experienced Segal taking in and remembering what he told her – so we can take back into ourselves our memories and feelings as thinkable and thought.

In 1993 the Segals had again moved, to share a house in north London with the family of their son Michael (a chemist who had by then become a senior civil servant). Paul Segal died in April 1996, and Hanna dedicated her next book, *Psychoanalysis, Literature and War*, to his memory. It includes a previously unpublished article that develops Bion's ideas about the importance of analysts taking in, understanding and appropriately conveying back to their patients their understanding of what is going on psychologically within them.[30] In it she quoted her one-time student Ronald Britton, whose furthering of our understanding of our inner–outer psychology is the subject of my last chapter.

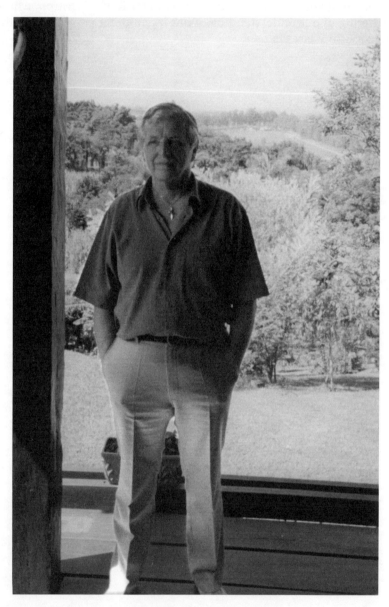

Ronald Britton in Brazil, 1998

10   Ronald Britton: Exclusions and Elegies

While Hanna Segal emphasizes acknowledging inner loss, beginning with the loss involved when, as babies, we first recognize our mothers' separateness from us, Ronald Britton emphasizes acknowledging the outer loss of being excluded from our parents' sexual involvement with each other. Perhaps it is his being a father (and also a grandfather) that leads Britton to draw attention to the place of both fathers and mothers in shaping our psychology. Perhaps it is also due to his being alert to what others – in particular his patients – make of him as a son, colleague, husband and father. Certainly he candidly acknowledges his concern with what his fellow Kleinians make of him. He has written of his 'publication anxiety'. He likens this anxiety in himself and other writers to fear of being attacked by onlookers envying the writer getting together with his readers. He likens this fear to Jean-Paul Sartre's account in *Being and Nothingness* of the fear of being reduced to a thing: of being witnessed watching through a keyhole two people making love.[1]

To guard against the voyeurism of others, especially as he still sees patients, Britton says little publicly about himself. He is also more scrupulous than many in protecting his patients from other people's voyeurism. He protects their anonymity by combining their different features and stories into fictional composites. And he supplements the result by also illuminating his theories with examples from poetry, notably that of Wordsworth and Rilke.

Wordsworthian beginnings[2]

Ronald Britton was born on 3 June 1932 in Lancaster, just south of Wordsworth's birthplace, Cockermouth, into a large extended family spread over north Lancashire, Cumbria and Yorkshire. He remembers his grandmothers as powerful figures: his mother's mother as a great source of domestic strength, and his father's mother as a 'mill girl' noted for saving her family from penury by starting a corner shop and going on to run several others. He describes his father as largely self-educated, very cultivated and well read, and a good musician. He ran a business with Ronald's mother, but this was disrupted by the Second World War, when he was away serving in the army.

Ronald, or 'Ron' as he is generally known, was their only child. He was very much the prototypical 'scholarship boy', he says. 'Since I was always dilatory as a student, exams have always saved me'. This included winning a scholarship, in 1943, to Lancaster's Royal Grammar School, which he attended until 1951. It was there, when he was eleven, that he first encountered the word 'atheist', from which he realized that his knowledge of God was a belief not a fact, a belief that he eventually rejected.[3] In his final year at school, when he was eighteen, he won the Princess Elizabeth Scholarship, which sent him with another boy from England to Southern Rhodesia (now Zimbabwe) for a few months. 'I suppose it was meant to form ties between Brits likely to be influential in either this country or over there', Britton explains. 'In fact it opened my eyes to racism in Africa and what I thought was bound to happen there fairly soon'.

On his return to England he started medical training at UCL and in April 1956 qualified as a doctor. On 17 June 1957 he married an American, Ritaclare Garlich, who had left her psychology studies in the United States to further develop her acting career at the Guildhall School of Music and Drama in London. Most of his friends, he says, were in literary studies or the theatre. In August that year he was called up for National Service, becoming a doctor in the army. His success in its postgraduate medical exams led to the army offering him training in whatever speciality he chose, provided he stayed in the army. He chose psychiatry, the area of medicine in which, from his earliest student days, he had always planned to specialize; in 1960 he was seconded to the National Hospital for Nervous Diseases, Queen's Square, London, and subsequently to various general psychiatry units (including Holloway Sanatorium in Virginia Water, Surrey). Later he went to the Maudsley Hospital in south-east London to train in child psychiatry, and subsequently to the Tavistock Clinic to learn psychotherapy, where his supervisors included Mattie Harris, Henry Ezriel and Pierre Turquet. By the time he left the army he had been promoted to a professorship in military psychiatry with senior tutor responsibilities for psychiatrists in both the army and the navy.

By then he was no longer the 'typical Maudsley organically minded psychiatric trainee':

> I was cured of that condition by the patients I met who reintroduced me to psychoanalysis by manifesting its theories in practice. I had read Freud at school and thought I knew better by the time I qualified as a doctor. But after a little time in psychiatry I was pushed by experience even further down the analytic road, eventually towards Kleinian thinking in an effort to understand what I was encountering.[4]

In 1969–71, during his army secondment to the Tavistock – where his teachers included Bob Gosling and David Malan – he went into analysis with the Kleinian analyst Claude Wedeles, beginning in 1970. In 1974 he was asked to apply for a job in the Tavistock's Children and Parents Department, where he became a consultant and of which he was chairman from 1976.

By then the Brittons had three children – Mark, Julie and Sophie. Ronald had also ended his analysis with Claude Wedeles when, in 1974, he began a ten-year analysis with Ruth Riesenberg Malcolm and started training at the Institute of Psycho-Analysis, where he was supervised by Betty Joseph and Hanna Segal. It was during this time that his first essays on psychoanalysis were published. They often dwelt on fathers.

Fathers

Britton prefaced his first psychoanalytic essay, 'The deprived child' (1978),[5] with the story of a father from Greek mythology – Tantalus, whom the gods punished by starving him and giving him food just out of reach for having killed and cooked his son and fed him to them. Britton used the story of Tantalus's cruelty to his son to highlight the fate of those who, deprived of feeling mothered inside, cruelly externalize and inflict their unhappiness on others. In another article, published in 1981, Britton drew attention to ways in which, for want of inwardly thinking through issues with which they are concerned, social workers and others in welfare agencies may find themselves acting out the feelings involved. He illustrated this inside-out process with the example of a boy with emotional and learning difficulties who had been abandoned by each of the agencies involved, just as the boy himself and his mother had been abandoned by his father.[6]

In 1981 Britton was elected to full membership of the British Psycho-Analytical Society after presenting an essay called 'The as-if personality' (see pp. 200–1 below). It was so highly commended by his assessors that he was temporarily paralysed, he says, at the prospect of writing anything else. During the resulting lull in his work he began attending the Wordsworth conferences held each summer in Grasmere, going there regularly from 1982 for the next twelve years.

In 1980 he had joined a workshop run by Betty Joseph, now regarded as one of the most important and influential Kleinians. Britton spoke about her psychoanalytic method to his fellow Kleinians in October 1983, the talk being called 'Some technical difficulties in speaking to the patient' (unpublished). That year he went on to publish a brief paper, 'Breakdown and reconstitution of the family circle', in which he drew attention to the 'paternal function' of childcare workers, warning them not to abdicate this function by looking to therapists to fulfil it instead.[7]

This was one of Britton's few papers on childcare. By 1983 his own children were nearly grown up. In 1984 he left the childcare work of the Tavistock's Children and Parents Department to devote himself to full-time private practice, working with adults as a psychoanalyst. The next year he became a training and supervising analyst to psychoanalytic students. Through his resulting teaching and clinical practice he arrived at his most important work: our pervasive flight from outer reality to inner 'Oedipal illusions'.

Oedipal illusions

In 1896 Freud famously related children's psychology to the myth of Oedipus killing his father and marrying his mother. In 1910 he somewhat revised his theory, stating that the 'Oedipus complex' starts with the boy, on the verge of puberty, learning about sexual intercourse. As a result, said Freud: 'He begins to desire his mother herself in the way with which he has recently become acquainted, and to hate his father anew as a rival who stands in the way of this wish'.[8] Britton spoke about this selfsame conflict of children with their fathers as well as with their mothers in a talk to his Kleinian colleagues in 1983. It represented something of a challenge to the then somewhat single-minded focus of many Kleinians on early mothering to the neglect of the place also occupied by fathers in our psychology. To 'placate the ancestors', as he put it,[9] Britton sought to demonstrate the continuity of his thesis with the early writings of Freud and Klein. He quoted their writings about fathers as well as mothers in discussing children's conflicts, upsets and persecutory and depressive anxieties at being excluded from their parents' sexual involvement with each other.

In a talk in Vienna in the summer of 1985 Britton highlighted the persistence of this upset into adulthood. He told the story, made up out of several of his patients' histories, of a middle-aged woman imagining her father brutally taking her mother away from her,[10] and herself taking revenge by cruelly attacking her mother for abandoning her for her father. She also sought concretely to get rid of her cruel imaginings – her 'bad thoughts', as she called them – by repeatedly and obsessively flushing the toilet, washing her hair and emptying rubbish down the garbage chute. But nothing can do away with the reality of our parents getting together sexually without us. She was accordingly endlessly compelled to repeat her obsessive rituals because they could never succeed in obliterating this reality. She tried and tried, but to no avail. For knowledge can never be undone. Once we know of our origin in our parents' sexual coupling we cannot unknow it. We cannot recover the innocence we had before knowing what we now know. Britton emphasized the point by quoting from Wordsworth's ode on the 'Intimations of Immortality': 'nothing can bring back the hour / Of splendour in the grass, of glory in the flower'.[11] Nevertheless we may seek to retreat from knowing what is outside by withdrawing into inner illusion. We may seek to avert unhappiness and depression about being excluded from our parents' sexual involvement with each other by illusorily keeping separate in our minds our knowledge of the mother who feeds us from our knowledge of the mother making love with the father. Britton gave the example of a patient who lyrically recalled sharing a meal with his girlfriend until she mentioned her former husband. At this he noticed a scar on her leg. It spoilt everything. He could no longer make love to her. Indeed he never saw her again, so much did her mentioning her husband evoke his wanting to attack his parents' sexual coupling, represented by the attack – the scar – on her leg.

Children too do not want to know. For example, a nine-year-old patient, Peter, had a resistance to knowing that led to his doing very badly at school. In therapy with Britton he retreated from knowing what was going on into a make-believe story. It concerned a primitive tribe. Peter called them 'the Wallies'. He was the all-powerful chief and sat on top of a mine shaft while his minions brought him food mined from below. After the first holiday break in his treatment, Peter added that the Wallies got rid of another character, 'Baron von Wally', for not feeding their chief. Perhaps, Britton commented, he felt he had similarly not been fed by him over the break. At this Peter began playing with two rulers, which he called ships – one British, the other American. He bumped their ends together. In doing so he crushed a little toy pug dog between them. He too had felt crushed by Britton getting together with an American colleague involved in working with his parents. He did not want to know. Hence his retreat into his story of himself as all-powerful chief being fed by the Wallies. Or so Britton said. At this Peter took up a toy camel. Then, referring to the camel's two humps, and to his older sister's new baby, he replied: 'Daniel, my baby, drinks from a cup. . . . He used to drink from my sister's tits but he did not like it so after about three weeks he gave it up, so now he drinks from a cup'.[12] He thereby emphasized that he could do without Britton over the three-week holiday break. He could feed himself, or be fed by his imagined Wally minions. He did not need Britton. Nor therefore did he need to know what Britton got up to with others – with his American colleague, for instance.

In his next article Britton drew attention to other ways in which children and adults variously maintain continuity between inner and outer reality, divide one from the other, or encapsulate inner within outer reality or the past within the present. Then he was invited by the Klein Trust to give the talk on Oedipal illusions (first presented privately to his fellow Kleinians in 1983) as a public lecture at UCL. Presenting this lecture in 1987, he argued that a major cause of adults and children dividing inner from outer reality is their feelings of deprivation, hatred, depression and loss at facing the outer reality of their parents and others getting together sexually without them. For some, attachment to one figure – in the first instance to the mother – is felt to be so precarious it cannot withstand the hatred unleashed by facing this figure's sexual involvement with someone else. Britton cited the case of a Miss A, who came into analysis after a psychotic breakdown in middle age. Having no sense of being mothered inside, Miss A could only retain a good image of her mother by restricting what she knew about her. This included refusing to take in the fact of her mother's sexual involvement with her father, so much did it signify her mother being unresponsive and dead to her. It was the same with Britton. She could not bear to know about him getting together with others, or about him having any other concern or thought even. It made her so desperate she protested and shouted, 'Stop that fucking thinking!'

Others find the idea of their mothers getting together with their fathers too depressing a loss to face. An example, said Britton, was a refugee patient who worked as a government scientist. He knew his parents lived together but he treated them as though they lived completely apart. He felt the same about Britton. He knew Britton was married. Indeed he knew Britton's wife. But he treated the two of them as though they had utterly separate lives. It was the same with his ideas: he kept them apart too. It had caused him learning difficulties when he was a child. Now he was grown up he still kept his ideas, things and people separate, fearing that if they came together someone might be killed. He had nightmares of a couple killing each other. He dreamt he might kill them. He dreamt a couple went off to the theatre together, leaving him alone with a dangerous, wild, *alter ego* figure who threatened to destroy everything, so upset and angry was he at their leaving him alone and going away together. He dreamt they went to the theatre of the absurd. It led him to think of plays performed in church, and to wonder whether they could include the word 'fuck', and whether he could ever face with Britton the idea of a couple sexually getting together without him.

Britton first spoke in 1983 about the impact of being excluded by others' sexual involvement with each other. But, as we have seen, he did not give a public talk on this subject until 1987, and it was not until 1989 that this talk was published.[13] By then Britton had begun giving monthly postgraduate seminars in Frankfurt. From 1990 he also became increasingly involved in giving lectures in London, in New York, Switzerland, Australia, California, Brazil and Moscow. In 1993, with John Steiner and Michael Feldman, he also started an annual residential conference for analysts from abroad at West Lodge, a hotel on the outskirts of London. Two years later, he was appointed chair of the British Psycho-Analytical Society's training analysts' committee. His articles and lectures came to be increasingly illustrated not only with fictionalized composites of his clinical cases, but also with quotations from poetry.

Patients and poets

In a public lecture published in 1992, Britton returned to the patient he had earlier described as getting rid of her cruel thoughts about her parents' sexual involvement with each other by obsessively flushing the toilet, washing her hair and emptying the rubbish. He said she also talked of wanting things inside cut out. 'If only someone would X-ray my mind', she yearned, 'and do an operation'.[14] But getting rid of what was bad inside made everything outside bad – so much so that she could not bear to travel beyond a short radius from her home in London. But she was also frightened of being stuck inside this small circumscribed area, just as in childhood she had been frightened of being stuck inside her mother, having learnt that hers had been a tubal pregnancy. She also

remembered being so frightened of being suffocated as a child confined with her mother in an air-raid shelter during the war that she
had tried to escape, only to be stopped by the warden at the door.
At this she had collapsed, lost all sensation, become paralysed, mute
and completely numb. She became terrified of this happening again,
of being buried alive, and of being suffocated by Britton. She was
also frightened that Britton might regard what she said as meaningless, or that he might forget and be stopped from taking in what she
said, just as she felt her father stopped her mother taking in what
she felt as a baby. In her mind her father was all bad, her mother all
good. She could not bear to know of them getting together. But keeping them apart left her mother a lifeless figure in whom she felt
entombed.

This conflict between life and death – and feeling entombed – is
not confined to patients. To highlight its ubiquity Britton quoted
Andrew Marvell's account of the soul complaining against the
entombing body:

> O, who shall from this Dungeon raise
> A soul enslaved so many ways?
> With bolts of bones, that fettered stands
> In feet, and manacled in hands.

Accused of being suffocating, the body replies that it cannot bear the
soul – its fears and feelings:

> the palsy shakes of fear;
> The pestilence of love does heat,
> Or hatred's hidden ulcer eat;
> Joy's cheerful madness does perplex,
> Or sorrow's other madness vex.[15]

Britton went on to publish an essay (based on his membership
paper of 1981 for the British Psycho-Analytical Society), in which
he illustrated the conflict of inner and outer reality with two clinical
examples.[16] The first involved a four-year-old, Tracy, who one
evening, together with her baby sister, witnessed their father violently
attacking their mother. The mother then tried to kill herself and was
taken to hospital. In therapy the next day, Tracy silently took out
some toy animals. She put a family of pigs on one side and various
wild animals on the other side of a barrier which she built between
them. She was afraid of the two getting mixed together – her bad
dreams and wild thoughts getting mixed up with what went on at
home, as her therapist put it. At this Tracy took the crocodile from
the wild animal side, and made it crawl over the barrier and attack

the mother and baby pig. At her next session, she reversed the process. She made a toy person climb over the barrier and join the wild animals, indicating interchange between the two realities – inside and out – the continuity between them having previously been disturbed by the trauma of what had happened at home.

Britton's second example involved a man who similarly climbed from one reality to the other, from outer to inner, wild to tame. He dreamt that tigers were attacking and eating people in Hyde Park. Feeling distressed and somehow responsible, he dreamt he went into the adjoining Kensington Gardens. But the tigers had also gone there. Fearful that they might attack and eat him, he got under the fence dividing the parks. Retelling his dream, he mused about the statue near the division between the two parks. What was it called? 'Peter Pan', he suddenly remembered. Then he added, 'Never-Never Land', alluding to his persistent hovering between inside and out in a never-never 'as-if' world, as Britton put it, of never committing himself whole-heartedly to knowing or believing what was going on.

Believing, Britton emphasized, gives 'psychic reality' to what we know. We may oscillate, as this patient did, between outer knowledge and inner belief. Or we may annihilate or suspend belief. Or we may answer it with a counter-belief. An example was a patient who, since childhood, believed that if her mother was out of sight she either no longer existed or was murderously involved with her father in the 'other room', as Britton called it. Terrified of these two imagined alternatives coming true, she answered them with a counter-belief that if she did not see her mother, or if her mother died, she would go blind.[17] She could not let her mother go. Her mother not being there left her feeling so insecure that she had to counter her knowledge of her being gone into another room with her father. In doing so, said Britton, she did away with the space needed for thinking and imagining.

Britton compared opening ourselves to this space – the 'other room' – to Keats's notion, also cited by Bion (see p. 129 above), of 'negative capability'. He said that the openness it involves depends on feeling securely mothered inside. If this is lacking we may do away with the openness, space and room needed for imagining, as this patient did. Or we may fill inner reality with a lie, as Blake's poem 'The Everlasting Gospel' (1818), describes:

> This Life's dim Windows of the Soul
> Distorts the Heavens from Pole to Pole
> And leads you to Believe a Lie
> When you see with, not thro', the Eye.[18]

Or we imagine ourselves getting in on the act. We intrude ourselves into the sexual involvement of our parents and others with each other. An example was Anna O, a patient of Freud's colleague Josef Breuer. Her hysterical breakdown, Britton pointed out, began when, nursing her sick father, she took her mother's place with him in their bedroom. In the same way she later took Breuer's wife's place with Breuer in imagining herself to be pregnant by him. One of Britton's patients similarly imagined taking his wife's place with him. She dreamt that she was a young girl having sex with Britton. He figured as an older man in her dream. In it she also figured as an older woman watching the scene from a cupboard.[19]

Alternatively, instead of thus watching and intruding ourselves into such scenes, we may face the reality of our being excluded from them. We may confront the truth of our exclusion from others' sexual involvement with each other. We may work through the accompanying joys and woes. But when the work is done we may resist ever facing the havoc again. According to Britton, Wordsworth did just this. After confronting his disillusion with the French Revolution, and after facing and contending with the turbulence of his affair with his French mistress, Annette Vallon, he settled for conventional married life. Wordsworth's 'Ode to duty', written in 1805, includes the following complacent homily:

> Me this uncharted freedom tires;
> I feel the weight of chance desires:
> My hopes no more must change their name,
> I long for a repose which ever is the same.[20]

Belief and imagination

Britton's book *Belief and Imagination*, published in 1998, highlights the hatred of outer reality impelling flight to inner illusion. The following passage, from Milton's *Paradise Lost*, evokes Satan's loathing of seeing a couple making love:

> Sight hateful, sight tormenting! Thus these two
> Imparadised in one another's arms
> The happier Eden, shall enjoy their fill
> Of bliss on bliss, while I to hell am thrust
> Where neither joy nor love, but fierce desire,
> Among our other torments not the least,
> Still unfulfilled with pain of longing pines.[21]

Suffering the pain and longing, Satan scorns and curses the couple:

> Live while ye may
> Yet happy pair; enjoy, till I return,
> Short pleasures, for long woes are to succeed.[22]

Milton's poem counters the outer heaven that the couple enjoys with the inner hell of Satan, Moloch and Beelzebub. This gang is akin to the inner Mafia which Rosenfeld (who supervised Britton after he qualified as an analyst) attributed to envious hatred of what we love and find good and depend upon in others (see pp. 106–8 above). In *Paradise Lost*, envious hatred of a loving couple drives Satan to quit what is outside for changeless timelessness and placelessness within:

> Farewell happy fields . . .
> Infernal world . . .
> Receive thy new possessor; one who brings
> A mind not to be changed by place or time.
> The mind its own place, and in itself
> Can make a heaven of hell, a hell of heaven
> Here we may reign secure, and in my choice
> To reign is worth ambition though in hell:
> Better to reign in hell, than serve in heaven.[23]

Or we may counter outer reality with unfounded inner hope and phantasy, as Christian does, according to Britton, in Bunyan's *The Pilgrim's Progress*. In this allegory, published in two parts in 1678 and 1684, Christian's first truth-seeking travelling companion, Faithful, is tried and executed by a court consisting of Lord Hate-good, and Messrs Envy, Blind-man, No-good, Malice, Love-lust, Live-loose, Heady, High-mind, Enmity, Liar, Cruelty, Hate-light and Implacable. Faithful gone, Christian replaces him with another travelling companion, Hopeful. In this, Britton found Christian similar to the hero of Voltaire's *Candide* (1759). Candide chooses as his travelling companion the absurdly hopeful Pangloss, with his 'all-is-the-best-in-the-best-of-all-possible-worlds' philosophy of 'pre-existing harmony' in a world of 'monads' or 'windowless souls' untouched by outer experience.

Similarly, in Britton's view, Blake retreated from outer reality into a vision of pre-existing inner harmony. Not that he did not take account of outer reality. In his *Songs of Experience* (1793), written at the time of the Terror in France, he noted the cruelty and corruption of Regency London, where:

> In every cry of every Man
> In every Infant's cry of fear,
> In every voice, in every ban,
> The mind-forg'd manacles I hear.[24]

But he also countered outer reality. In *The Book of Los* (1795), Blake evoked retreat into inner bliss:

> When Love & Joy were adoration,
> And none impure were deem'd:
> Not Eyeless Covet,
> Nor Thin-lip'd Envy,
> Nor Bristled Wrath,
> Nor Curled Wantonness.[25]

In another poem from the *Songs of Experience* (series of 1801), Blake, as the poem's narrator, yearns for his mother never to have brought him out of inner heaven into outer hell. He berates her:

> Thou, Mother of my Mortal part,
> With cruelty didst mould my Heart,
> And with false self-deceiving tears
> Didst bind my Nostrils, Eyes, & Ears
> Didst close my Tongue in senseless clay,
> And me to Mortal Life betray.[26]

He prayed to be liberated: 'Death of Jesus set me free'.[27] Longing for freedom from outer bodily mortality – and from the outward-facing science and reason of Bacon, Locke and Newton – he willed himself in *Jerusalem* (1804–20), to make an alternative world from within: 'I must Create a System or be enslav'd by another Man's. / I will not Reason & Compare: my business is to Create'.[28]

Or we might flee from outer reality into inner romance, a point made by Britton with Emily Brontë's *The Prisoner* as example. Brontë's poem evokes an innocent girl – 'soft and mild / As sculptured marble saint or slumbering, unweaned child' – saved from unjust punishment by an idealized paternal figure, Lord Julian; it also describes the pain of awakening from inner romance into outer reality. Britton used the same stanza as Tustin did to illustrate this point (see p. 168 above):

> Oh, dreadful is the check – intense the agony
> When the ear begins to hear and the eye begins to see;
> When the pulse begins to throb, the brain to think again,
> The soul to feel the flesh and the flesh to feel the chain![29]

While Brontë, Blake and Milton described fleeing from the painfulness of outer reality, others describe steadfastly facing it. Britton felt that the young Wordsworth was particularly notable in this respect, citing how, at the age of twenty-eight, Wordsworth had uncompromisingly faced the sadness of what goes on both inside and out:

> I have learned
> To look on nature, not as in the hour
> Of thoughtless youth, but hearing oftentimes
> The still, sad music of humanity.[30]

In 1798 Wordsworth abandoned Annette Vallon, the mother of his child, and resolutely faced her unhappiness in his poem 'The Ruined Cottage':

> her poor hut
> Sunk to decay: for he was gone, whose hand
> At the nipping of October frost
> Closed up each chink.[31]

He was mindful of the 'presence of loss', as Britton described it: 'a *presence* which in his youth provided him with a direct physical experience of bliss and later, after its disappearance, interfused all things . . . like the incarnation of Christ, followed after his disappearance by Pentecost and the "inspiration" of the Holy Ghost'.[32] Britton's book goes on to discuss Wordsworth's *The Prelude* (1799 version), finding in it the origin of our adult 'creative sensibility' in what is outside us, depicted as stemming from our internalizing our outward attachment to our mothers:

> blest the babe
> Nursed in his mother's arms, the baby who sleeps
> Upon his mother's breast, who, when his soul
> Claims manifest kindred with an earthly soul,
> Doth gather passion from his mother's eye.
> Such feelings pass into his torpid life
> Like an awakening breeze, and hence his mind . . .
> Subjected to the discipline of love,
> His organs and recipient faculties
> Are quickened, are more vigorous; his mind spreads,
> Tenacious of the forms which it receives. . . .
> From this beloved presence – there exists
> A virtue which irradiates and exalts
> All objects through all intercourse of sense.[33]

Rilke outside in

It is above all through his account of the poetry of Rilke that Britton's *Belief and Imagination* most movingly conveys the process of internalizing outer reality and its irradiation from within. Rilke depicted this outer–inner movement particularly eloquently in the course of composing *The Duino Elegies*. In an early elegy he described his resistance to bringing together his inner and outer worlds. Britton assimilated them to the subjective and objective, maternal and paternal poles of the Oedipal triangle. In the words of Rilke's translator, we resist bringing outer and inner together lest one vanish into the other:

> Though someone may tell us:
> 'Yes, you've entered my bloodstream, the room the whole springtime
> is filled with you' . . . what does it matter? he can't contain us,
> we vanish inside him and around him . . .[34]

The elegy evokes our warding off outer reality. This begins with the mother fending off and hiding outer reality from her baby:

> you shielded him just by placing
> your slender form between him and the surging abyss?
> How much you hid from him then.[35]

But, this is futile. Warding off outer reality does not protect the inner world. Instead it leaves it a place of dread:

> who could ward off,
> who could divert, the floods of origin inside him?
> . . . dreaming . . .
> he was caught up
> and entangled in the spreading tendrils of inner event
> already twined into patterns, into strangling undergrowth, prowling
> bestial shapes.[36]

Rilke completed the third elegy, in which these lines occur, in 1913. After a long pause, in June 1914 he sent Lou Andreas Salomé (his lover who later became a close confidante and correspondent of Freud) a poem called *Turning Point*. In it Rilke announced, in effect, that the crucial issue is not to ward off but to take in and transform with love what is seen outwardly within. Of seeing the outward world he now wrote:

> Long he had won it by looking.
> Stars would fall on their knees
> under his strenuous up-glance . . .
> Towers he would gaze at so.[37]

But, wrote Britton, the world wants to be loved, not just gazed at. In Rilke's words:

> Work of seeing is done,
> now practise heart-work
> on those images captive within you; for you
> overpowered them only: but now do not know them.
> Look, inward man, look at your inward maiden,
> her, the laboriously won
> from a thousand natures, at her the
> being till now only
> won, never yet loved.[38]

But again the mother interferes. In an unpublished poem written in October 1915 Rilke complained:

> Oh, misery, my mother tears me down.
> Stone upon stone I'd laid, towards a self
> and stood like a small house, with day's expanse around it,
> Now comes my mother, comes and tears me down.[39]
> . . .
> Birds overhead more lightly fill my space.
> Strange dogs can sense it . . .
> Only my mother does not know
> My oh how slowly incremented face.[40]

His mother might not want to know, but Rilke was now ready to know and to countenance bringing what is outside in. The next month he returned to *The Duino Elegies*. In the fourth elegy, known as 'The Marionette Elegy', Rilke insisted on facing what is outside:

> I *must* stay seated, must
> wait before the puppet stage, or rather,
> gaze at it so intensely that at last,
> to balance my gaze, an angel has to come and
> make the stuffed skins startle into life.[41]

Facing the outer world – including facing death, represented by the inanimate figures of the puppet stage – an angel startles it into inner life. 'The angel', Rilke explained, 'is that creature in whom the transformation of the visible into the invisible, which we are accomplishing, appears already consummated'.[42] It is the means by which what is externally visible is transformed into what is invisible within us. Our task, wrote Rilke, is

> to stamp this provisional, perishing earth into ourselves so deeply, so painfully and passionately, that its being may rise again, 'invisibly', in us. We are the bees of the Invisible. . . . The *Elegies* show us this at work, this work of the continual conversion of the dear visible and tangible into the invisible vibration and agitation of our own nature.[43]

Rilke's account of the transformation of what is outward into what is invisible within us brings me to the end of Britton's insights into the importance of this outer–inner process. It also brings me to the end of my book's account of the revolution he and others have brought about in using psychoanalysis, poetry and art to advance our understanding of the inside-out as well as the outside-in dynamic of our psychology. Where, to conclude, does it lead us?

Conclusion: Further Integrations

Melanie Klein herself as well as her colleagues, analysands, students and followers today have done an enormous amount to highlight the interaction of inner and outer reality shaping both our dreams and our waking life from infancy onwards. They have thereby crucially illuminated the ways in which imagination and phantasy, creativity and inner life animate our everyday outer reality.

But Kleinians have been concerned with more than psychological health. They have extended their concerns to embrace psychological ills and unhappiness – the greed, envy and hatred with which we attack what is best and most loving, loved and good within and beyond us. Through unflinchingly confronting the dualities of love and hate in health and distress, Kleinians have enormously extended our understanding of the psychology of both children and adults, including the ills done them by neurosis, hypochondria, depression, anorexia, autism and schizophrenia.

Kleinians emphasize that recovery from these ills, and psychological health generally, depends on integrating and bringing together inner and outer reality. Ronald Britton has described the life-enhancing transformation that can result from what we take in from outside being irradiated by what Rilke called an 'angel' within us. Freud, too, emphasized that health depends on bringing together our inner- and outer-directed unconscious and conscious minds. Melanie Klein took this further through extending Freud's discoveries about the inner unconscious world of our dreams in also investigating the dream-like phantasies of waking life. She drew attention, much more than Freud, to ways in which our inner psychology is peopled by images of those with whom we are outwardly involved. She argued that health depends on our overcoming paranoid-schizoid preoccupation with inner persecutory anxieties. It also depends on overcoming the obstacles of omnipotence, denial, idealization and projective identification that prevent us from loving and experiencing inner and outer figures in our lives as loving, loved and good. It depends in the first instance on early experience of the mother as loving and loved, free from phantasies of greedily emptying or enviously spoiling everything loving and loved within her. Internalizing her as an object of love and goodness provides the kernel for further integration.

Summarizing further, I have sought to show how Klein's colleague and friend Susan Isaacs detailed ways in which children's phantasies mediate and integrate their inner and outer reality. Meanwhile Joan Riviere illuminated aspects of our inner world, including envy and depression, and ways in which they can become concealed by outer masquerades of femininity and masculinity, jealousy, dominance and control. Adrian Stokes extended these insights to aesthetics; his writings on the value of ballet and art show how our inner and outer worlds can be integrated through stabilizing externally what is psychologically fraught within us.

Following the Second World War medically qualified psychoanalysts – notably Herbert Rosenfeld, Wilfred Bion and Hanna Segal – pioneered the extension of Klein's ideas to treating, healing and integrating the inner–outer divisions involved in schizophrenia. Just as Stokes described movement from inside out to outside in, they described movement from inside out in the transference of patients of their inner world on to the outer figure of the analyst. They also described the countertransference impact on analysts of being made the outward repository of their patients' inward phantasies.

Esther Bick and Frances Tustin advanced the insights of Klein and Bion in emphasizing the importance of infant observation and how this can alert therapists and others not only to the inner world of adults and children, but to flight from lack of inner integration through clinging to outer surfaces and shapes. Ronald Britton has explored another flight – from unhappiness at being excluded from the sexual involvement of others, initially that of our parents, into retreat to a divided-off world of inner illusion.

The division of inner and outer reality is a major cause of the ills for which people seek help from therapists and psychoanalysts. Hence the emphasis of psychoanalysts – and notably of Kleinians – on bringing these two realities together. In his book *Psychic Retreats* (1993), the London-based Kleinian John Steiner emphasized that health depends on taking back into ourselves and thereby integrating what we otherwise split off and externalize into others. This is increasingly being emphasized by psychoanalysts not only in England but also in mainland Europe, North and South America, South Africa, India and Australia.

This in turn involves further integrations. Psychoanalysts and psychoanalytically minded psychotherapists, counsellors and others – once bitterly divided, as they were at the time of the British Psycho-Analytical Society's wartime discussions – are now increasingly coming together in adopting Klein's ideas. Particularly important in this process has been their development by Wilfred Bion. He emphasized the need to experience others containing our feelings if we are to internalize them as contained within ourselves. Increasingly this inner–outer perspective is also integrating psychoanalysis with politics, with feminist, gay and lesbian and with anti-racist causes, from which psychoanalysts have often in the past distanced themselves and cut themselves off. Lastly, and largely because of its increasing Kleinianism, psychoanalysis is becoming integrated with other disciplines in the sciences and humanities, including spirituality and religion to which it was once bitterly opposed. The book *Emotion and Spirit* (1984) by Neville Symington, the husband of Esther Bick's infant observation student Joan Cornwall, argues that psychoanalysis is akin to religion in seeking to bring together our inner and outer worlds to achieve what is good.

But what is good? This question is central to the integrations promoted by Kleinianism. It can be answered only in the context in which we find ourselves here, now and in the future, faced with the task of integrating the inner and outer realities explored by the women and men whose work and lives, together with those of their child and adult patients, I have described in this book. In doing so I very much hope I have conveyed some of the inspiration I have found in learning about them, and about the inside-out revolution they began, and which is even now continuing and expanding in psychoanalysis and psychology across the world.

Notes

Dates of lectures given at psychoanalytic congresses are reflected in the text; original dates of publication are given in the notes immediately after the author's name, where applicable, followed by publication details of a later collection.

Abbreviations

CA   *Childhood and After* by Susan Isaacs, London: Routledge & Kegan Paul, 1948

CWAS   *The Critical Writings of Adrian Stokes*, 4 vols, London: Thames & Hudson, 1978

EG   *Envy and Gratitude: The Writings of Melanie Klein*, vol. III, London: Hogarth, 1975

JCP   *Journal of Child Psychotherapy*

IJPA   *International Journal of Psycho-Analysis*

LGR   *Love, Guilt and Reparation: The Writings of Melanie Klein*, vol. I, London: Hogarth, 1975

SE   *The Standard Edition of the Complete Psychological Works of Sigmund Freud*, 24 vols, translated and edited by James Strachey, London: Hogarth, 1953–74

Introduction

1   In using the term 'phantasy' I adopt its Kleinian meaning, first systematically theorized by Susan Isaacs. She emphasized that 'phantasy'

refers specifically to the products of the unconscious. However she and other Kleinians have used the term to denote both conscious and unconscious phenomena. And it is in this interchangeable sense that I use the term in this book.

2 H. Segal (1979) *Klein*, London: Fontana, p. 55.
3 I deplore the use of the male pronoun to refer generically to babies and others, regardless of their sex. Nevertheless I adopt this convention both because it is less cumbersome than using its various alternatives, and because it provides a means of distinguishing babies and children from their primary caregivers who, given the continuing unequal sexual division of childcare, are mostly women.

1 Melanie Klein: Discovering Inner Reality

1 Details of Klein's life are based on H. Segal (1973) *Introduction to the Work of Melanie Klein*, London: Hogarth; H. Segal (1979) *Klein*, London: Fontana; P. Grosskurth (1986) *Melanie Klein*, London: Hodder & Stoughton; M. Klein (n.d.) *Autobiography*, London: Wellcome Institute; and J. Sayers (1991) *Mothering Psychoanalysis*, London: Penguin Books.
2 M. Klein (1921) 'The development of a child', in M. Klein (1975) *Love, Guilt and Reparation (LGR)*, London: Hogarth, pp. 1–53 (3, n. 1).
3 Ibid., p. 28.
4 Ibid., pp. 33–4.
5 Ibid., p. 43.
6 M. Klein (1923) 'The role of the school in the libidinal development of the child', in *LGR*, pp. 59–76.
7 M. Klein (1925) 'A contribution to the psychogenesis of tics', in *LGR*, pp. 106–27.
8 M. Klein (1926) 'The psychological principles of early analysis', in *LGR*, pp. 128–38; M. Klein (1932) *The Psycho-Analysis of Children*, London: Hogarth.
9 Klein, *Psycho-Analysis of Children*, pp. 17, 23.
10 Ibid., pp. 26–8.
11 Klein, *LGR*, pp. 128–38, and *Psycho-Analysis of Children*.
12 Klein, *Psycho-Analysis of Children*, p. 49, n. 2.
13 A. Strachey (1925), letter of 11 January, in P. Meisel and W. Kendrick (1986) *Bloomsbury/Freud: The Letters of James and Alix Strachey 1924–1925*, London: Chatto & Windus, p. 180.
14 A. Freud (1927) 'Introduction to the technique of the analysis of children', in A. Freud (1946) *The Psycho-Analytical Treatment of Children*, London: Imago.
15 M. Klein (1927) 'Symposium on child-analysis', in *LGR*, pp. 139–69.
16 M. Klein (1928) 'Early stages of the Oedipus conflict', in *LGR*, pp. 186–98.

17 M. Klein (1929) 'Infantile anxiety situations reflected in a work of art and in the creative impulse', in *LGR*, pp. 210–18 (210).

18 M. Klein (1930) 'The importance of symbol-formation in the development of the ego', in *LGR*, pp. 219–32.

19 Ibid., p. 227.

20 M. Klein (1935) 'A contribution to the psychogenesis of manic-depressive states', in *LGR*, pp. 262–89.

21 M. Klein (1940) 'Mourning and its relation to manic-depressive states', in *LGR*, pp. 344–69 (368).

22 M. Klein (1945) 'The Oedipus complex in the light of early anxieties', in *LGR*, pp. 370–419; M. Klein (1961) *Narrative of a Child Analysis*, London: Hogarth.

23 W. R. D. Fairbairn (1944) 'Endopsychic structure considered in terms of object relationships', in W. R. D. Fairbairn (1952) *Psychoanalytic Studies of the Personality*, London: Routledge, pp. 82–132.

24 M. Klein (1946) 'Notes on some schizoid mechanisms', in M. Klein (1975), *Envy and Gratitude (EG)*, London: Hogarth, pp. 1–24 (7).

25 M. Klein (1955) 'On identification', in *EG*, pp. 141–75.

26 M. Klein (1957) 'Envy and Gratitude', in *EG*, pp. 176–235 (202).

27 M. Klein (1959) 'Our adult world and its roots in infancy', in *EG*, pp. 247–63.

2 Susan Isaacs: Children's Phantasies

1 Biographical details are drawn from J. Rickman (1950) 'Obituary: Susan Sutherland Isaacs', *IJPA*, vol. 31, pp. 279–85; D. Gardner (1969) *Susan Isaacs*, London: Methuen; L. Smith (1985) *To Understand and to Help: The Life and Work of Susan Isaacs (1885–1948)*, Cranbury, NJ: Associated University Presses; A. Wooldridge (1994) *Measuring the Mind*, Cambridge: Cambridge University Press; M. Milner (1998) personal communication, 13 March.

2 Anon. (1948), 'Dr Susan Isaacs, CBE', *Nature*, 4 December, p. 881.

3 Gardner, *Isaacs*, p. 31.

4 S. Isaacs (1934) 'Rebellious and defiant children', in S. Isaacs (1948) *Childhood and After (CA)*, London: Routledge & Kegan Paul, pp. 23–35 (34).

5 Ibid., p. 35.

6 Gardner, *Isaacs*, p. 21.

7 Ibid., p. 37.

8 Ibid.

9 J. Brever and S. Freud (1893) 'On the physical mechanism, of hysterical phenomena', *SE2*, pp. 3–27.

10 S. Brierley (1918) 'Analysis of the spelling process', *Journal of Experimental Pedagogy*, vol. 4, pp. 239–54; S. Brierley (1921), *An Introduction to Psychology*, London: Methuen.

11 S. Brierley (1920) 'The present attitude of employees to industrial psychology', *British Journal of Psychology*, vol. 10, pp. 210–27; S. Brierley

(1921) 'Science and human values in industry', *The Co-operative Educator*, January.

12   E. Lawrence (1960) 'Foreword', in N. Isaacs, *A Brief Introduction to Piaget*, New York: Agathon Press.

13   S. Brierley (1923) 'A note on sex differences', *British Journal of Medical Psychology*, vol. 3, pp. 288–308 (300).

14   Rickman, 'Obituary', p. 279.

15   D. Lampe (1959) *Pyke: The Unknown Genius*, London: Evans.

16   W. Van der Eyken and B. Turner (1969) *Adventures in Education*, London: Allen Lane.

17   Miss Ogilvie later became a housemother (known as Toe) at another progressive school, Dartington, Devon, started by Dorothy and Leonard Elmhirst, to which several Malting House pupils also went. Like Pyke, Leonard Elmhirst was determined that children should not suffer the miseries he had suffered at school, in his case from his Bakewell prep school, where the headmaster was Mr Storrs Fox. See M. Young (1982) *The Elmhirsts of Dartington*, London: Routledge & Kegan Paul.

18   S. Payne (1952) 'Obituary: Dr. John Rickman', *IJPA*, vol. 33, pp. 54–60.

19   P. Meisel and W. Kendrick (1986) *Bloomsbury/Freud: The Letters of James and Alix Strachey 1924–1925*, London: Chatto & Windus, p. 136.

20   Rickman, 'Obituary', p. 281.

21   Meisel and Kendrick, *Bloomsbury/Freud*, p. 205.

22   S. Isaacs (1930) *Intellectual Growth in Young Children*, London: Routledge & Kegan Paul, pp. 188–9.

23   N. Isaacs (1927) 'Appendix A: Children's "why" questions', 'Appendix B: Education and science', in S. Isaacs, ibid., pp. 291–349, 350–4.

24   Anon. (1927) 'Education and science', *Nature*, 23 July, pp. 105–7.

25   S. Isaacs (1929) review of *The Child's Conception of the World* by J. Piaget, *Mind*, vol. 38, pp. 506–13; S. Isaacs (1929) 'A critical review of Piaget', *Journal of Genetic Psychology*, vol. 36, pp. 597–609; J. Piaget (1931) review of *Intellectual Growth in Young Children* by S. Isaacs, *Mind*, vol. 40, pp. 137–60; S. Isaacs (1931) review of *The Child's Conception of Causality* by J. Piaget, *Mind*, vol. 40, pp. 89–93; S. Isaacs (1934) review of *The Moral Judgement of the Child* by J. Piaget, *Mind*, vol. 43, pp. 85–99.

26   Isaacs, *Intellectual Growth*, pp. 182–3.

27   Ibid., p. 106.

28   B. Russell (1931) *The Scientific Outlook*, London: Allen & Unwin, p. 186.

29   S. Isaacs (1933) *Social Development in Young Children*, London: Routledge, pp. 19, 13.

30   Ibid., p. 210.

31   Ibid., pp. 113, 114–15.

32   Ibid., pp. 121, 122.

33   Ibid., pp. 143, 158, 142.

34   Ibid., p. 170.

35   Ibid., pp. 172, 173.
36   Ibid., p. 93.
37   Ibid., pp. 94, 99, 106.
38   S. Isaacs (1928) 'The mental hygiene of the pre-school child', in *CA*, pp. 1–9.
39   S. Isaacs (1929) 'Privation and guilt', in *CA*, pp. 10–22.
40   Anon. (1948) 'Obituary', *The Times*, 13 October, p. 6.
41   S. Isaacs (1929) *The Nursery Years*, London: Routledge & Kegan Paul, pp. 24, 92.
42   S. Isaacs (1932) *The Children We Teach*, London: University of London Press.
43   J. Pole (1948) 'Susan Isaacs', *New Statesman and Nation*, 23 October, p. 350.
44   A third Malting House book, *Individual Histories*, was planned but did not materialize.
45   Gardner, *Isaacs*, p. 168.
46   See letters to Bill Currie from Susan Isaacs (dated January and May 1934), currently owned by Sue Isaacs-Elmhirst.
47   Gardner, *Isaacs*, p. 101.
48   Isaacs, 'Rebellious and defiant children'.
49   S. Isaacs (1935) 'Property and possessiveness', in *CA*, pp. 36–46.
50   S. Isaacs (1935) 'Bad habits', *IJPA*, vol. 16, pp. 446–54.
51   H. R. Hamley, S. Isaacs and others (1937) *The Educational Guidance of the School Child*, London: Evans Brothers.
52   I. Hellman (1990) *From War Babies to Grandmothers*, London: Karnac.
53   The pamphlets, issued in 1937–8, were called *Concerning Children* and consisted of 'Weaning' by F. Shepherd, 'Concentration in young children' by M. Guttridge, 'The first two years' by S. Isaacs, 'School reports' by G. Swane, 'Friendships in adolescence' by S. Yates, 'The beginnings of reading and writing' by F. Roe, 'The baby who does not conform to rules' by F. Shepherd, 'Independence in adolescence' by S. Yates, 'Imagination and play in children by R. Griffiths and 'Play in the infant school' by E. Boyce; from M. Milner (1938) *The Human Problem in Schools*, London: Methuen, p. 314.
54   The series included Milner's *Human Problem in Schools*. See also J. Sayers (1989) 'Marion Milner', *BPS Psychology of Women Newsletter*, no. 3, pp. 3–13; A. Karpf (1998) 'Journey to the centre of the mind', *The Guardian*, 3 June, p. 21.
55   S. Isaacs (1938) 'Recent advances in the psychology of young children', in *CA*, pp. 74–88.
56   S. Isaacs (1939) 'Criteria for interpretation', in *CA*, pp. 109–21.
57   S. Isaacs (1943) 'An acute psychotic anxiety occurring in a boy of four years', in *CA*, pp. 143–85 (145).
58   S. Isaacs (1940) 'Temper tantrums in early childhood in their relation to internal objects', in *CA*, pp. 129–42.
59   P. Grosskurth (1986) *Melanie Klein*, London: Hodder & Stoughton, pp. 243–4.
60   S. Isaacs (1939) 'Modifications of the ego through the work of analysis', in *CA*, pp. 89–108 (102).

61 S. Isaacs (1939) 'A special mechanism in a schizoid boy', in *CA*, pp. 122–8.
62 S. Isaacs, ed., with the co-operation of S. Clement Brown and R. H. Thouless (1941) *The Cambridge Evacuation Survey*, London: Methuen.
63 S. Isaacs (1942) 'Children of Great Britain in wartime', in S. M. Gruenberg, ed., *The Family in a World at War*, New York: Harper, pp. 159–60.
64 S. Isaacs (1943) 'The nature and function of phantasy', in P. King and R. Steiner (1991) *The Freud–Klein Controversies 1941–1945*, London: Routledge & Kegan Paul, pp. 276–7.
65 Ibid., p. 308.
66 Isaacs, *Nursery Years*, p. 96.
67 S. Isaacs (1937) 'The educational value of the nursery school', in *CA*, pp. 47–73; see also Anon. (1948), in *The Times*, 13 October, p. 6.
68 Gardner, *Isaacs*, p. 135.
69 P. Heimann and S. Isaacs (1943) 'Regression', in King and Steiner, eds, *Freud–Klein Controversies*, p. 690.
70 S. Isaacs (1945) 'Notes on metapsychology as process theory', *IJPA*, vol. 26, pp. 58–62.
71 S. Isaacs (1945) 'Fatherless children', in *CA*, pp. 186–207.
72 Anon. (1948), in *Nature*, 4 December, p. 881.
73 S. Isaacs (1945) 'Children in institutions', in *CA*, pp. 208–36 (234).
74 Grosskurth, *Klein*, p. 368.
75 Anon. (1948), in *The Times*, 13 October, p. 6.
76 S. Isaacs (1948) 'The nature and function of phantasy', *IJPA*, vol. 29(2), pp. 73–97 (88).

3 Joan Riviere: Gendered Masquerades

1 Biographical details are drawn from J. Riviere (1905–19) selections from appointments books, London: Institute of Psycho-Analysis Library, (CRC/FO1/01); J. Strachey, P. Heimann, and L. Monro (1963) 'Obituary: Joan Riviere (1883–1962)', *IJPA*, vol. 44, pp. 228–35; P. Grosskurth (1986) *Melanie Klein*, London: Hodder & Stoughton; M. Milner (1988) personal communication, 30 September; A. Hughes (1991) *The Inner World and Joan Riviere*, London: Karnac; L. Appignanesi and J. Forrester (1992) *Freud's Women*, London: Weidenfeld & Nicolson; A. Hughes (1992) 'Letters from Sigmund Freud to Joan Riviere (1921–1939)', *IJPA*, vol. 19, pp. 265–84; A. Hughes (1997) 'Personal experience – professional interests: Joan Riviere and femininity', *IJPA*, vol. 78, pp. 899–911; M. Milner (1998) personal communication, 13 March.
2 Strachey, *IJPA*, vol. 44, p. 228.
3 Hughes, *IJPA*, vol. 78, p. 906.
4 Ibid., pp. 900, 906.
5 Strachey, *IJPA*, vol. 44, p. 228.
6 K. West (1958) *Inner and Outer Circles*, London: Cohen & West, p. 26.

7   30 October 1918, in V. Brome (1982) *Ernest Jones: Freud's Alter Ego*, London: Caliban Books, p. 116.

8   J. Riviere (1920) 'Three notes', in Hughes, *Inner World*, pp. 46–9.

9   Hughes, *IJPA*, vol. 19, p. 268.

10 22 January 1922, in R. A. Paskauskas (1993) *The Complete Correspondence of Sigmund Freud and Ernest Jones*, Cambridge: Harvard University Press, pp. 453–4.

11 23 March 1922, in Paskauskas, *Correspondence*, p. 464.

12 11 May 1922, in ibid., p. 475.

13 4 June 1922, in ibid., pp. 483–7 (484).

14 S. Freud (1923) *The Ego and the Id. SE19*, pp. 12–66 (49).

15 24 August 1922, in Pauskauskas, *Correspondence*, p. 499.

16 10 September 1922, in Hughes, *IJPA*, vol. 19, p. 271.

17 3 October 1922, in Hughes, *Inner World*, pp. 36, 39.

18 30 January 1923, in Hughes, *IJPA*, vol. 19, p. 271.

19 J. Riviere (1921–2) review of *Psychoanalyis* by R. Hingley, in Hughes, *Inner World*, pp. 71–3 (71).

20 J. Riviere (1921–2) review of *Dreams and the Unconscious* by C. W. Valentine, in Hughes, ibid., pp. 74–6 (76).

21 J. Riviere (1921–2) review of *The Technique of Psycho-Analysis* by D. Forsyth, in Hughes, ibid., pp. 64–70 (70).

22 J. Riviere (c.1920–1) 'The theory of dreams', in Hughes, ibid., pp. 54–8 (57).

23 J. Riviere (1923) review of J. Strachey's translation of *Group Psychology and the Analysis of the Ego* by S. Freud, in Hughes, ibid., pp. 60–1 (61).

24 2 July 1923, in Hughes, *IJPA*, vol. 19, p. 274.

25 J. Riviere (1924) review of *The Psychology of Dress* by F. Alvah Parsons, in Hughes, *Inner World*, p. 77.

26 J. Riviere (1924) 'A castration symbol', in Hughes, ibid., pp. 51–2.

27 J. Riviere (1924) 'The castration complex in a child', in Hughes, ibid., pp. 49–51.

28 J. Riviere (1924) 'Phallic symbolism', in Hughes, ibid., p. 52.

29 J. Riviere (1929) 'Womanliness as a masquerade', in Hughes, ibid., pp. 90–101; This has been cited approvingly, for example by S. Case (1993) 'Toward a butch-femme aesthetic', in H. Abelove, M. Barale and D. Halperin, eds, *The Lesbian and Gay Studies Reader*, London: Routledge, pp. 294–306. For a critique of recent feminist failure to note the racism of Riviere's article, see J. Walton (1995) 'Re-placing race in (white) psychoanalytic discourse', reprinted in E. Abel, B. Christian and H. Moglen (1997) *Female Subjects in Black and White*, Berkeley: University of California Press, pp. 223–50.

30 J. Riviere (1927) 'Symposium on child analysis', in Hughes, *Inner World*, pp. 80–7 (84).

31 9 October 1927, in Hughes, *IJPA*, vol. 19, p. 280.

32 18 October 1927, in Paskauskas, *Correspondence*, p. 635.

33 22 October 1927, ibid., pp. 635–6.

34 9 September 1928, in Hughes, *IJPA*, vol. 19, p. 281.

35 L.-A. Sayers (1998) personal communication, 30 May. See also A. Motion (1986) *The Lamberts*, London: Chatto & Windus.

36 J. Riviere (1930) 'Magical regeneration by dancing', in Hughes, *Inner World*, pp. 53–4.

37 P. King and R. Steiner (1991) *The Freud–Klein Controversies 1941–1945*, London: Routledge, p. xix.

38 A. Phillips (1988) *Winnicott*, London: Fontana.

39 J. Riviere (1932) 'Jealousy as a mechanism of defence', in Hughes, *Inner World*, pp. 104–15.

40 J. Riviere (1934) review of *New Introductory Lectures on Psycho-Analysis* by S. Freud, in Hughes, ibid., pp. 118–31.

41 J. Riviere (1936) 'A contribution to the analysis of the negative therapeutic reaction', in Hughes, ibid., pp. 134–53 (144).

42 S. Freud 11923) *The Ego and the Id*, *SE19*.

43 P. Heimann (1963) 'Obituary: Joan Riviere', *IJPA*, vol. 44, pp. 230–3 (232).

44 J. Riviere (1936) 'On the genesis of psychical conflict in earliest infancy', in Hughes, *Inner World*, pp. 272–300 (279).

45 Ibid., p. 286.

46 J. Riviere (1937) 'Hate, greed and aggression', in Hughes, ibid., pp. 167–205 (169, 170); also in M. Klein and J. Riviere (1937), *Love, Hate and Reparation*, London: Hogarth.

47 Ibid., p. 173.

48 Ibid., p. 176.

49 Ibid., p. 181.

50 Ibid., p. 183.

51 J. Riviere (1937) review of *An Autobiographical Study* by S. Freud, in Hughes, *Inner World*, pp. 156–66.

52 J. Riviere (1939) 'An intimate impression', in Hughes, ibid., pp. 208–12 (212).

53 11 June 1944, National Archives of Canada at Ottawa Clifford Scott papers.

54 Milner (1998) personal communication, 13 March.

55 H. Segal (1991) 'Foreword', in Hughes, *Inner World*, pp. xi–xiv.

56 J. Riviere (1945) 'The bereaved wife', in Hughes, ibid., pp. 214–26.

57 J. Riviere (1948) review of *The Question of Lay Analysis* by S. Freud, in Hughes, ibid., pp. 228–30.

58 J. Riviere (1952) 'General introduction' to M. Klein et al. (1952) *Developments in Psycho-Analysis*, in Hughes, ibid., pp. 233–69 (234, 269).

59 J. Riviere (1952) 'The unconscious phantasy of an inner world reflected in examples from literature', in Hughes, ibid., pp. 302–30 (309).

60 Ibid., p. 319.

61 Ibid., p. 320.

62 Ibid., p. 321.

63 Ibid., p. 326.

64 J. Riviere (1952) 'The inner world in Ibsen's *Master Builder*', in Hughes, ibid., pp. 332–47.

65 J. Riviere (1958) 'A character trait of Freud's', in Hughes, ibid., pp. 350–4 (351).
66 Ibid., p. 353.
67 King and Steiner, eds, *Freud–Klein Controversies*, p. xix.
68 H. Segal (1986) 'Hanna Segal', in E. H. Baruch and L. J. Serrano (1988) *Women Analyze Women*, New York: New York University Press, pp. 241–55.
69 Heimann, *IJPA*, vol. 44, p. 232.
70 Segal, in Hughes, *Inner World*, p. xiv.

4 Adrian Stokes: Ballet and Art

1 E. Rhode (1973) 'Memories of Adrian Stokes', *The Listener*, 13 December, pp. 812–15.
2 Unless otherwise indicated biographical details are drawn from A. Stokes (1947) *Inside Out*, in *CWASII*, pp. 139–82; A. Stokes (1951) *Smooth and Rough*, in *CWASII*, pp. 213–56; Rhode, 'Memories'; R. Wollheim (1980) 'Adrian Stokes', *PN Review*, vol. 7(1), pp. 31–7; P. Robinson (1981) *With All the Views*, Manchester: Carcanet; R. Read (1982) 'Adrian Stokes', *Adrian Stokes 1902–72: A Retrospective*, London: Arts Council, pp. 51–7; R. Wollheim (1986) 'Stokes', in Lord Blake and C. S. Nicholls, eds (1986) *Dictionary of National Biography 1971–1980*, Oxford: Oxford University Press, pp. 809–10; R. Read (1995) 'Art criticism versus poetry', *Comparative Criticism*, vol. 17, pp. 133–60; A. Angus (1998) personal communication, 22 September; R. Wollheim (1998) personal communication, 22 June; A. Angus (1999) personal communication, 21 June; N. Glover (1999) *Psychoanalytic Aesthetics*, London: Process Press; and R. Read (1999) personal communication, 5 January and 6 August.
3 D. Stokes (1929) *The Last Step (An Essay on the Philosophy of Personality)*, London: Simpkin, Marshall.
4 Stokes, *Inside Out*, p. 142.
5 Ibid., p. 146.
6 Ibid., p. 150.
7 A. Stokes (n.d.) *London Childhood*, quoted in Robinson, *With All the Views*, p. 54.
8 Stokes, *Inside Out*, p. 170.
9 Stokes, *Smooth and Rough*, p. 227.
10 A. Stokes (1922) 'Dilemma', *Oxford Fortnightly Review*, 10 February, pp. 330–2; R. Read (1980) 'Freudian psychology and the early work of Adrian Stokes', *PN Review*, vol. 7(1), pp. 37–40.
11 Stokes, *Inside Out*, pp. 156, 157.
12 P. Quennell (1976) *The Marble Foot*, p. 142, quoted in P. Ziegler (1998) *Osbert Sitwell*, London: Chatto & Windus, p. 164.
13 Rhode, 'Memories', p. 813.
14 J. Middleton Murray, 'Introduction', in A. Stokes (1925) *The Thread of Ariadne*, London: Kegan Paul, Trench, Trübner, p. vii.

15   S. Bann (1988) 'Adrian Stokes', in N. Segal, ed., *Freud in Exile*, New Haven: Yale University Press.

16   A. Stokes (1926) *Sunrise in the West*, London: Kegan Paul, Trench, Trübner.

17   A. Stokes (1930) 'Pisanello', *Hound and Horn*, vol. 4, no. 1, Oct–Dec, pp. 5–25, reprinted in *Comparative Criticism* (1995), vol. 17, pp. 161–207 (164).

18   Ibid., pp. 164, 165.

19   Read, *Comparative Criticism*, vol. 17, p. 149.

20   A. Stokes (1933) review of *The Psycho-Analysis of Children* by M. Klein, *The Criterion*, vol. 9 (April), pp. 527–30.

21   A. Stokes (1933) 'Mr Ben Nicholson's painting', *The Spectator*, 27 October, reprinted in *CWASI*, pp. 307–8.

22   N. Stungo (1999) 'Writers block', *The Observer*, 17 January, p. 4.

23   A. Stokes (1934) *Stones of Rimini*, reprinted in *CWASI*, pp. 181–301 (184, 235). The book included material from A. Stokes (1929) 'The sculptor Agostino di Duccio', *The Criterion*, vol. 9, no. 34, pp. 44–60, and A. Stokes (1933) 'From the Tempio', *The Criterion*, vol. 13, no. 50, pp. 7–24. It was reviewed by Ezra Pound (1934) in *The Criterion*, vol. 13, no. 52, pp. 495–7.

24   Stokes, *Stones of Rimini*, p. 183.

25   Ibid., p. 252.

26   Ibid., p. 300.

27   Ibid., p. 265.

28   P. Smith (1980) 'Adrian Stokes and Ezra Pound', *PN Review*, vol. 7(1), pp. 51–2.

29   Read, *Comparative Criticism*, vol. 17, pp. 133–60.

30   A. Stokes (1934) *To-Night the Ballet*, London: Faber, p. 23.

31   Ibid., p. 26.

32   Ibid., p. 39.

33   Ibid., p. 78.

34   Wollheim, in *DNB*.

35   A. Stokes (1935) *Russian Ballets*, London: Faber, p. 68.

36   Ibid., p. 164. The painting formerly known as *The Flagellation* is now generally accepted as a depiction of *The Dream of St Jerome* (Galleria Nazionale, Urbino).

37   For further details see B. Laughton (1986) *The Euston Road School*, Aldershot: Scolar Press.

38   A. Stokes (1937) 'Mr Ben Nicholson at the Lefèvre Galleries', *The Spectator*, March, reprinted in *CWASI*, pp. 315–16 (316).

39   A. Stokes (1937) *Colour and Form*, reprinted in *CWASII*, pp. 7–83 (13).

40   Ibid., p. 21.

41   Ibid., p. 18.

42   See, for example, A. Stokes (1930) 'Painting, Giorgione and Barbaro', *The Criterion*, vol. 9(36), pp. 482–500; A. Stokes (1949) *Art and Science*, reprinted in *CWASII*, pp. 183–212.

43   Stokes, in *CWASII*, p. 71.

44   Ibid., p. 75.

45   For more on the relation between Stokes and Auden, see L. Stone-bridge (1998) *The Destructive Element*, London: Macmillan.
46   A. Stokes (1945) *Venice*, London: Faber, p. 12, n. 1.
47   Ibid., p. 62.
48   A. Stokes (1945) 'Concerning art and metapsychology', *IJPA*, vol. 26(3–4), pp. 177–9 (177).
49   Stokes, *Inside Out*, p. 141.
50   Ibid., p. 166.
51   A. Stokes (1947) *Cézanne*, reprinted in *CWASII*, pp. 257–72 (268, 269).
52   A. Stokes (1951) 'A note on abstract or symphonic ballet', *Adelphi*, February, pp. 44–6; A. Stokes (1951) 'Piero della Francesca', *The Spectator*, March.
53   Personal communication, 13 July 1999.
54   A. Stokes (1952) 'A study of Tintoretto', *The Spectator*, January; A. Stokes (1956) *Raphael*, London: Faber, reprinted in *CWASIII*, 273–88; A. Stokes (1958) *Monet*, London: Faber, reprinted in *CWASIII*, pp. 289–303.
55   A. Stokes (1955) *Michelangelo*, reprinted in *CWASIII*, pp. 7–76 (27).
56   Ibid., pp. 53, 54.
57   A. Stokes (1955) 'Form in art', in M. Klein et al. (1977), eds, *New Directions in Psycho-Analysis*, London: Karnac, pp. 406–20 (411).
58   Ibid p. 418, n. 1.
59   A. Stokes (1973) *A Game that Must be Lost: Collected Papers*, ed. E. Rhode, Cheadle Hulme: Carcanet Press. The book includes the following Imago Group papers: 'Listening to clichés', 'Psycho-analytic reflections on the development of ball games', 'On being taken out of oneself', 'Primary process, thinking and art' and 'Psycho-analysis and our culture'.
60   A. Stokes (1956) review of *Art and Visual Perception* by R. Arnheim. 'Seeing as action', *Encounter*, 6 March, pp. 91–3.
61   A. Stokes (1958) *Monet*, reprinted in *CWASII*, pp. 289–303 (294).
62   A. Stokes (1958) *Greek Culture and the Ego*, reprinted in *CWASIII*, pp. 77–141 (126).
63   A. Stokes (1960–1) 'The impact of architecture', *British Journal of Aesthetics*, reprinted in *CWASIII*, pp. 189–205.
64   A. Stokes (1961) *Three Essays on the Painting of Our Time*, reprinted in *CWASIII*, pp. 143–84 (158).
65   Ibid., p. 182.
66   Ibid., p. 151.
67   A. Stokes (1962) 'Coldstream and the sitter', reprinted in *CWASIII*, pp. 185–88 (188).
68   A. Stokes (1962) 'On resignation', *IJPA*, vol. 43, pp. 175–81.
69   Wollheim, *PN Review*, vol. 7(1), p. 36.
70   A. Stokes (1963) *Painting and the Inner World*, reprinted in *CWASIII*, pp. 207–59 (249).
71   A. Stokes (1964) review of *Our Adult World and Other Essays* by M. Klein, *IJPA*, vol. 45, pp. 131–4.

72   A. Stokes (1964) review of *Introduction to the Work of Melanie Klein* by H. Segal, *New Statesman*, vol. 67, p. 367.

73   A. Stokes (1964) review of *Monastic Architecture in France* by J. Evans, *British Journal of Aesthetics*, vol. 4, no. 4, p. 371.

74   A. Stokes (1964) 'Herbert Read', *British Journal of Aesthetics*, vol. 4, pp. 195–6.

75   A. Stokes (1964) 'Living in Ticino, 1947–50', *Art and Literature*, vol. 1, pp. 314–20.

76   Stokes (1965) also wrote an introduction to the exhibition catalogue, *Lawrence Gowing*, London, Marlborough Fine Art.

77   G. Burn (1965) 'Profile', *Arts Review*, vol. 17(1), p. 2.

78   A. Stokes (1965) *Venice*, London: Duckworth.

79   A. Stokes (1965) *The Invitation in Art*, reprinted in *CWASIII*, pp. 261–342.

80   A. Stokes (1966) 'On being taken out of one's self', *IJPA*, vol. 47, pp. 523–30.

81   A. Stokes (1966) 'The image in form', *British Journal of Aesthetics*, vol. 4, pp. 46–64.

82   A. Stokes (1967) *Reflections on the Nude*, reprinted in *CWASIII*, pp. 301–42 (313).

83   A. Stokes (1969) 'Reminiscences', *Ben Nicholson: A Studio International Special*, p. 14.

84   A. Stokes (1967) review of *Turner* by L. Gowing, *British Journal of Aesthetics*, vol. 7, pp. 207–8; A. Stokes (1971) review of *Freud* by R. Wollheim, *The Listener*, 29 April, p. 554.

85   A. Stokes (1972) 'The future and art', *Studio International*, vol. 184, reprinted in Stokes, *Collected Papers*, ed. Rhode, pp. 146–60 (151).

86   R. Read (1998) personal communication, 7 December.

87   R. Wollheim (1999) personal communication, 15 July.

88   A. Stokes (n.d.) *Schizophrenic Girl*, in Robinson, *With All the Views*, pp. 124–5 (124). A selection of Stokes's poetry can be found, together with that of Geoffrey Grigson and Edwin Muir, in *Penguin Modern Poets 23*, and in Robinson.

89   R. Read (1998) personal communication, 14 December.

90   A. Stokes (1972) 'We are the animals we keep', quoted in Robinson, *With All the Views*, p. 161.
     Very movingly his daughter, Ariadne to whom he had also written another poem quoted in this chapter, wrote after his death: 'I had been reading for a little and I have been watching television. How is Philip and how is Ian, hey, and I want to play football with him and I am sorry that Daddy is not alive. And I know that he was born and I know the year won't come again. I want to go to see Mrs Hart again who taught me ballet lessons didn't she, I remember.'

91   Wollheim, in *DNB*, p. 810.

92   See, for example, D. Carrier (1980) 'Adrian Stokes and recent American painting', *PN Review*, vol. 7(1), pp. 50–1; P. Fuller (1985) *Images of God*, London: Chatto; L.-A. Sayers (1993) 'She might pirouette on a daisy and it would not bend', in H. Thomas, ed., *Dance, Gender*

and Culture, London: Macmillan; R. Read (1993) 'Art criticism versus art history', *Art History*, vol. 16(4), pp. 499–540; R. Read (1998) 'Art today: Stokes, Pound, Freud and the word-image opposition', *Word & Image*, vol. 14(3), pp. 227–52.

5   Herbert Rosenfeld: Schizophrenics and Gangsters

1   Biographical details are drawn from H. Rosenfeld (1963) 'Notes on the psychopathology and psycho-analytic treatment of schizophrenia', in H. Rosenfeld (1965) *Psychotic States*, London: Hogarth, pp. 155–68; H. Rosenfeld (1977) 'Personal experiences in treating psychotic patients', in K. A. Frank, ed., *The Human Dimension in Psychoanalytic Practice*, New York: Grune & Stratton, pp. 29–48; H. Rosenfeld (1987) *Impasse and Interpretation*, London: Routledge; H. Segal and R. Steiner (1987) 'Obituary: H. A. Rosenfeld (1910–1986)', *IJPA*, vol. 68, pp. 415–19; A. Rosenfeld (1998) personal communication, 22 May; A. Heyne (1998) personal communication, 8 June.

2   H. Rosenfeld (1947) 'Analysis of a schizophrenic state with depersonalisation', in Rosenfeld, *Psychotic States*, pp. 13–33; see also Rosenfeld, 'Notes'.

3   Quoted in S. Freud (1911) 'Psycho-analytic notes on an autobiographical account of a case of paranoia', *SE12*, p. 70.

4   H. Rosenfeld (1949) 'Remarks on the relation of male homosexuality to paranoia', in Rosenfeld, *Psychotic States*, pp. 34–51; H. Rosenfeld (1950) 'Notes on the psychopathology of confusional states in chronic schizophrenias', in Rosenfeld, *Psychotic States*, pp. 52–62.

5   H. Rosenfeld (1952) 'Notes on the psycho-analysis of the superego conflict in an acute schizophrenic patient', in Rosenfeld, *Psychotic States*, pp. 63–103; H. Rosenfeld (1952) 'Transference-phenomena and transference-analysis in an acute catatonic schizophrenic patient', in Rosenfeld, *Psychotic States*, pp. 104–116.

6   H. Rosenfeld (1954) 'Considerations regarding the psycho-analytic approach to acute and chronic schizophrenia', in Rosenfeld, *Psychotic States*, pp. 117–27; see also Rosenfeld, 'Notes'; H. Rosenfeld (1964) 'An investigation into the need of neurotic and psychotic patients to act out during analysis', in Rosenfeld, *Psychotic States*, pp. 200–16.

7   H. Rosenfeld (1964) 'An investigation into the need of neurotic and psychotic patients to act out during analysis', in Rosenfeld, *Psychotic States*, pp. 200–16; H. Rosenfeld (1964) 'The psychopathology of drug addiction and alcoholism', in Rosenfeld, *Psychotic States*, pp. 217–42.

8   H. Rosenfeld (1964) 'The psychopathology of hypochondriasis', in Rosenfeld, *Psychotic States*, pp. 180–99.

9   H. Rosenfeld (1968) 'Notes on the negative therapeutic reaction', paper read to the British Psycho-Analytic Society and to the Meninger Clinic, Topeka.

10 H. Rosenfeld (1971) 'A clinical approach to the psychoanalytic theory of the life and death instincts', *IJPA*, vol. 52, pp. 169–78; see also Rosenfeld, *Impasse and Interpretation*.

11 H. Rosenfeld (1964) 'Object relations of the acute schizophrenic patient in the transference situation', *Psychiatric Research Reports of the American Psychiatric Association*, vol. 19, pp. 54–68; see also H. Rosenfeld (1981) 'On the psychopathology and treatment of psychotic patients', in J. S. Grotstein, ed., *Do I Dare Disturb the Universe?*, London: Karnac, pp. 168–79; Rosenfeld, *Impasse and Interpretation*.

12 H. Rosenfeld (1978) 'Notes on the psychopathology and psychoanalytic treatment of some borderline patients', *IJPA*, vol. 59, pp. 215–21.

6 Wilfred Bion: Group and Individual Analysis

1 Biographical details are based principally on Bion's own writings, most of which were published posthumously, edited by his widow, Francesa Bion: *War Memoirs (1917–19)*, London: Karnac 1997; *The Dream* (1975), *The Past Presented* (1977) and *The Dawn of Oblivion* (1979) in W. Bion (1991) *A Memoir of the Future*, London: Karnac; *The Long Week-End 1897–1910* (1982), London: Free Association Books; and *All My Sins Remembered* (1985), Abingdon: Fleetwood Press. I have also drawn on Anon. (1985) 'Bion: An appreciation', in M. Pines, ed., *Bion and Group Psychotherapy*, London: Tavistock, pp. 386–9; G. Bléandonu (1990) *Wilfred Bion*, London: Free Association Books 1994; F. Bion (1980) 'Envoi', in Bion, *Sins Remembered*; F. Bion (1982) 'Foreword', in Bion, *Long Week-End*; F. Bion (1994) 'The days of our years', talk given in Toronto; F. Bion (1997) Introduction, in *Taming Wild Thoughts*, London: Karnac; F. Bion (1997) 'Random reflections on Bion', Turin; F. Bion (1997) personal communication, 30 October; F. Bion (1999) further discussions.

2 W. Bion (1977–9) *Bion in New York and São Paulo*, Perthshire: Clunie Press, 1980, p. 10.

3 Bion, *Long Week-End*, p. 32.

4 Letter of 1963, quoted in Bion, *Sins Remembered*, p. 173.

5 Bion, *Long Week-End*, p. 45.

6 Ibid., p. 46.

7 Ibid., p. 106.

8 Ibid., p. 195.

9 Ibid., pp. 248, 249.

10 Ibid., p. 264.

11 Bion, *Memoir of the Future*, p. 423.

12 Bion, *War Memoirs*, p. 198.

13 Founded as the Hampstead Football Club in 1866, the Harlequins remain one of England's top rugger clubs, based since 1906 in Twickenham. My thanks to Steve Uglow for this information.

14   H. Dicks (1970) *Fifty Years of the Tavistock Clinic*, London: Routledge, p. 10.

15   Bion, *Sins Remembered*, p. 218.

16   Anon. (1981) *Old Stortfordian Newsletter*, January, pp. 387–8.

17   J. S. Grotstein (1981) 'Wilfred R. Bion', in J. S. Grotstein, ed., *Do I Dare Disturb the Universe?* London: Karnac, pp. 1–35.

18   F. Bion, 1997, personal communication.

19   W. R. Bion (1940) 'The "war of nerves"', in E. Miller, ed., *The Neuroses in War*, London: Macmillan, pp. 180–200.

20   W. R. Bion (1946) 'The leaderless group project', *Bulletin of the Menninger Clinic*, vol. 10, pp. 77–81.

21   T. Harrison and D. Clarke (1992) 'The Northfield experiments', *British Journal of Psychiatry*, vol. 160, pp. 698–708; T. Harrison (1999) *Bion, Rickman, Foulkes and the Northfield Experiments*, London: Jessica Kingsley.

22   W. R. Bion and J. Rickman (1943) 'Intra-group tensions in therapy', *Lancet*, vol. 2, pp. 218–21, reprinted in W. R. Bion (1961) *Experiences in Groups*, New York: Ballantine, pp. 3–17 (10).

23   Bion, *Bulletin of the Menninger Clinic*, vol. 10, p. 80.

24   Bion, *Sins Remembered*, p. 70.

25   E. Trist (1985) 'Working with Bion in the 1940s', in Pines, ed., *Bion and Group Psychotherapy*, pp. 1–46.

26   W. R. Bion (1951) 'Group dynamics', *IJPA*, vol. 33(2), reprinted in Bion, *Experiences in Groups*, pp. 134–5.

27   F. Bion, in Bion, *Sins Remembered*, p. 239.

28   W. R. Bion (1950) 'The imaginary twin', in W. R. Bion (1967) *Second Thoughts*, London: Heinemann, pp. 3–22 (5).

29   W. R. Bion (1953) 'Notes on the theory of schizophrenia', in Bion, *Second Thoughts*, pp. 23–35.

30   W. R. Bion (1955) 'Language and the schizophrenic', in M. Klein, P. Heimann and R. E. Money-Kyrle, eds (1955) *New Directions in Psycho-Analysis*, London: Tavistock, pp. 220–39 (224).

31   W. R. Bion (1956) 'Development of schizophrenic thought', in Bion, *Second Thoughts*, pp. 36–42.

32   W. R. Bion (1957) 'Differentiation of the psychotic from the non-psychotic personalities', in Bion, *Second Thoughts*, pp. 43–64 (53).

33   W. R. Bion (1957) 'On arrogance', in Bion, *Second Thoughts*, pp. 86–92.

34   W. R. Bion (1958) 'On hallucination', in Bion, *Second Thoughts*, pp. 65–85.

35   W. R. Bion (1959) 'Attacks on linking', in Bion, *Second Thoughts*, pp. 93–109.

36   W. R. Bion (1960) 'Dream-work and alpha', in W. Bion (1994) *Cogitations*, London: Karnac, p. 186.

37   Letter of 27 March 1960, quoted in Bion, *Sins Remembered*, p. 134; see also Bion, *Memoir of the Future*, p. 622; Bion, *Cogitations*, p. 333.

38   Reproduced in Bion, *Sins Remembered*, p. 189.

39   W. R. Bion (1967) 'Notes on memory and desire', in E. Bott Spillius, ed., *Melanie Klein Today*, London: Routledge, vol. 2, pp. 17–21.

40 Letter of 21 December 1817 from John Keats to George and Thomas Keats, quoted in W. R. Bion (1970) *Attention and Interpretation*, London: Tavistock, p. 125.
41 Ibid., p. 129.
42 W. R. Bion (1967) 'Synopsis and notes', in Bion, *Cogitations*, pp. 254–92.
43 F. Bion, 'Days of our years'.
44 M. Milner (1998) personal communication, 13 March.
45 Trist, in Pines, ed., *Bion and Group Psychotherapy*, pp. 1–46.
46 Bion, *Cogitations*, p. 376.
47 F. Bion, 'Days of our years'.
48 W. R. Bion (1973–4) *Brazilian Lectures*, London: Karnac, 1990, p. 54.
49 Ibid., p. 135.
50 W. R. Bion (1975) 'Brasilia', in W. R. Bion (1994) *Clinical Seminars and Other Works*, London: Karnac, pp. 3–139.
51 W. R. Bion (1976) 'Emotional turbulence', in *Clinical Seminars*, pp. 295–305.
52 W. R. Bion (1977) *Two Papers: The Grid and Caesura*, London: Karnac, 1989, p. 12.
53 W. Bion (1960) 'Alpha', 24 February, in *Cogitations*, pp. 141–3.
54 Bion, *Two Papers*, p. 18.
55 W. Bion (1978) 'São Paulo', in *Clinical Seminars*, pp. 141–240 (175).
56 W. Bion (1979) 'Making the best of a bad job', in *Clinical Seminars*, pp. 321–31.
57 Bion, *Memoir of the Future*, p. 162.
58 W. Bion (1974) letter to Julian, in Bion, *Sins Remembered*, p. 219.

7   Esther Bick: Infant Observation

1 Biographical details are based on M. Harris (1983) 'Esther Bick (1901–1983)', *JCP*, vol. 9(2), pp. 101–2; A. Hughes (1984) 'Notes for a meeting in Turin in memory of Bick', 15 July; B. Joseph (1984) informal address in memory of Mrs Bick, Tavistock Clinic, May; J. Magagna (1987) 'Three years of infant observation with Mrs Bick', *JCP*, vol. 13(1), pp. 19–39; E. Wedeles (1998) personal communication, 9 June; S. Mancia (n.d.) interview with E. Bick; P. Lussana (n.d.) unpublished essay; I. Menzies Lyth (1998) personal communication, 26 June; R. Riesenberg Malcolm (1999) personal communication, 17 February; and J. Symington (1995) 'Mrs Bick and infant observation', Second European Colloquium on Infant Observation, Toulouse.
2 Mancia, interview, p. 3.
3 I. Hellman (1990) *From War Babies to Grandmothers*, London: Karnac, p. 3.
4 Mancia, interview, p. 4.
5 Magagna, *JCP*, vol. 13(1), p. 19.
6 Mancia, interview, p. 11.
7 S. Isaacs-Elmhirst (1997) 'A scientific turn of mind', in T. Mitrani and

J. Mitrani, eds, *Encounters with Autistic States*, San Francisco: Jason Aronson, pp. 209–12.

8 Symington, lecture, p. 2.

9 E. Bick (1964) 'Notes on infant observation in psycho-analytic training', *IJPA*, vol. 45, pp. 558–66 (562).

10 Symington, lecture, p. 8.

11 E. Bick (1953) 'Anxieties underlying phobia of sexual intercourse in a woman', National Archives of Canada at Ottawa, Clifford Scott papers, MG31J30, vol. 57.19.

12 I. Wittenberg (1997) 'Beginnings', in S. Reid, ed., *Developments in Infant Observation*, London: Routledge, pp. 19–32.

13 M. Rustin (1987) 'Introduction', in M. Harris, ed., *Collected Papers of Martha Harris and Esther Bick*, Perthshire: Clunie Press, pp. ix–xii.

14 E. Bick (1961) 'Child analysis today', in M. Harris, ed., *Collected Papers*, pp. 104–13.

15 My thanks to Ann Stokes, now Ann Angus, for telling me about Ariadne's treatment for the purposes of this book.

16 E. Bick (1968) 'The experience of the skin in early object-relations', *IJPA*, vol. 49, pp. 484–86 (485).

17 D. Meltzer (1974) 'Adhesive identification', in D. Meltzer (1994) *Sincerity and Other Works*, London: Karnac, pp. 335–50 (344).

18 E. Bick (1986) 'Further considerations on the function of the skin in early object relations', *British Journal of Psychotherapy*, vol. 2(4), pp. 292–9 (298).

19 Mrs Bick must have misremembered, says Ann Angus in a letter of 13 July 1999: 'Adrian would *never* have said there was nothing to see in Florence'.

20 Magagna, *JCP*, vol. 13(1), p. 19.

8   Frances Tustin: Anorexia and Autism

1 Biographical details are drawn from F. Tustin (1981) 'A modern pilgrim's progress', *JCP*, vol. 7, pp. 175–9; F. Tustin (1984) 'The growth of understanding', *JCP*, vol. 10(2), pp. 137–48, revised in F. Tustin (1986) *Autistic Barriers in Neurotic Patients*, London: Karnac, pp. 33–47; S. Spensley (1995) *Frances Tustin*, London: Routledge; V. Hamilton (1998) correspondence; and G. Tustin (1998) correspondence.

2 Spensley, *Tustin*, p. 6.

3 Ibid., p. 7.

4 F. Tustin (1951) *A Group of Juniors*, London: Heinemann, pp. 74–5.

5 Spensley, *Tustin*, p. 17.

6 Tustin, *JCP*, vol. 7, p. 175.

7 For further details of Margaret's case, see F. Tustin (1958) 'Anorexia nervosa in an adolescent girl', *British Journal of Medical Psychology*, vol. 31(3–4), pp. 184–200; F. Tustin (1986) *Autistic Barriers in Neurotic Patients*, London: Karnac.

8 V. Sinason (1998) personal communication, 31 March.

9   F. Tustin (1963) 'Two drawings occurring in the analysis of a latency child', *JCP*, vol. 1(1), pp. 41–6.

10 V. Hamilton (1995) 'Foreword', in F. Tustin (1972) *Autism and Childhood Psychosis*, London: Karnac, pp. xi–xiv, xx.

11 For further details of John's case, see F. Tustin (1966) 'A significant element in the development of autism', *JCP*, vol. 7, pp. 53–67; Tustin, *Autism*; Tustin (1981) *Autistic States in Children*, London: Routledge, revised edition 1992; Tustin, *Autistic Barriers*; and Tustin (1990) *The Protective Shell in Children and Adults*, London: Karnac.

12 E. Bick (1968) 'The experience of the skin in early object-relations', *IJPA*, vol. 49, pp. 484–6.

13 For further details of David's case, see F. Tustin (1969) 'Autistic processes', *JCP*, vol. 2(3), pp. 23–39; Tustin, *Autism*; Tustin, *Autistic States*; Tustin, *Autistic Barriers*.

14 V. Hamilton (1997) 'The analysis of a 9-year-old girl with learning disabilities', in T. Mitrani and J. Mitrani, eds, *Encounters with Autistic States*, San Francisco: Jason Aronson, pp. 83–110 (84).

15 For further details of Peter's case, see Tustin *Autistic States*; and Tustin, *Protective Shell*.

16 A. Newman (1994) obituary letter, *The Guardian*, 21 December, p. 15.

17 Tustin, *Autistic States*, p. 176.

18 Spensley, *Tustin*, p. 7.

19 M. Rhode (1995) 'A tribute to Frances Tustin', *JCP*, vol. 21(2), pp. 153–66.

20 T. B. Brazelton (1969) *Infants and Mothers*, New York: Dell, p. 137, quoted in F. Tustin (1983) 'Thoughts on autism with special reference to a paper by Melanie Klein', *JCP*, vol. 9(2), pp. 119–31, revised in Tustin, *Autistic Barriers*, pp. 48–66.

21 J. Van Buren (1997) 'Themes of being and non-being in the work of Frances Tustin and Jacques Lacan', in Mitrani and Mitrani, eds, *Autistic States*, pp. 195–207.

22 Tustin, *JCP*, vol. 2(3), p. 31.

23 Tustin, *Autistic Barriers*, p. 144.

24 Ibid., p. 224.

25 Ibid., p. 235.

26 Ibid., p. 236.

27 Ibid., p. 302.

28 Ibid., p. 296.

29 Ibid., p. 203.

30 Ibid., p. 200.

31 Ibid., p. 198.

32 Ibid., p. 14, see also Tustin, *Autistic States*, p. 232.

33 Tustin, *Protective Shell*, p. 12. See also F. Tustin (1991) 'Revised understandings of psychogenic autism', *IJPA*, vol. 72(4), pp. 585–91; F. Tustin (1994) 'The perpetuation of an error', *JCP*, vol. 20(1), pp. 3–23.

34 Tustin, *Protective Shell*.

35 See, for example, S. Baron-Cohen (1989) 'The autistic child's theory of mind', *JCP*, vol. 30(2), pp. 285–97.
36 J. L. Mitrani (1997) 'Preface', in Mitrani and Mitrani, eds, *Autistic States*, pp. xv–xx (xix).
37 Hamilton, in Mitrani and Mitrani, eds, *Autistic States*, pp. 83–110.
38 My thanks to Sheila Spensley, letter of 15 July 1999, for this information.

9 Hanna Segal: Symbolism and Psychosis

1 Biographical details are drawn from E. H. Baruch and L. J. Serrano, eds, *Women Analyze Women*, New York: University Press, 1988, pp. 241–55; D. Bell (1997) *Reason and Passion: A Celebration of the Work of Hanna Segal*, London: Duckworth; and H. Segal (1998) interview, 26 October.
2 Baruch and Serrano, eds, *Women Analyze Women*, p. 242.
3 Bell, *Reason and Passion*, p. 3.
4 H. Segal (1952) 'A psycho-analytic approach to aesthetics', in H. Segal (1981) *The Work of Hanna Segal*, New York: Jason Aronson, pp. 185–206 (189).
5 Ibid., p. 195.
6 Ibid., p. 196.
7 Ibid., p. 203.
8 H. Segal (1950) 'Some aspects of the analysis of a schizophrenic', in Segal, *Work*, pp. 101–20 (104).
9 H. Segal (1953) 'A necrophilic phantasy', in Segal, *Work*, pp. 165–71.
10 H. Segal (1956) 'Depression in the schizophrenic', in Segal, *Work*, pp. 121–9 (127).
11 H. Segal (1957) 'Notes on symbol formation', in Segal, *Work*, pp. 49–65.
12 H. Segal (1958) 'Fear of death', in Segal, *Work*, pp. 173–81 (176).
13 Ibid., p. 178.
14 H. Segal (1964) *Introduction to the Work of Melanie Klein*, London: Hogarth, pp. 87–8.
15 H. Segal (1972) 'Role of child analysis in the general psychoanalytic training', *IJPA*, vol. 53, pp. 157–61.
16 H. Segal (1972) 'A delusional system as a defence against the re-emergence of a catastrophic situation', in H. Segal (1997) *Psycho-analysis, Literature and War*, London: Routledge, pp. 49–63 (50).
17 Ibid., p. 55.
18 H. Segal (1974) 'Delusion and artistic creativity', in Segal, *Work*, pp. 207–16.
19 W. Golding (1964) *The Spire*, London: Faber, pp. 210–11.
20 H. Segal (1977) 'Psychoanalysis and freedom of thought', in Segal, *Work*, pp. 217–27.
21 J. Conrad (1917) *The Shadow Line*, London: Penguin, 1986, p. 45.

22   H. Segal (1987) 'Silence is the real crime', in Segal, *Psychoanalysis*, pp. 143–56.
23   H. Segal (1991) *Dream, Phantasy and Art*, London: Routledge, p. 87.
24   H. Segal (1992) 'The achievement of ambivalence', *Common Knowledge*, vol. 1, pp. 92–104.
25   H. Segal (1995) 'Hiroshima, the Gulf War and after', in Segal, *Psychoanalysis*, pp. 157–68. For examples of patients refusing to face, or indulging phantasies of nuclear annihilation, see H. Segal (1993) 'On the clinical usefulness of the concept of death instinct', *IJPA*, vol. 74, pp. 55–62.
26   H. Segal (1994) 'Salman Rushdie and the sea of stories', in Segal, *Psychoanalysis*, pp. 133–42.
27   H. Segal (1978) 'On symbolism', in Segal, *Psychoanalysis*, pp. 41–8.
28   H. Segal (1994) 'Phantasy and reality', in Segal, *Psychoanalysis*, pp. 27–40.
29   Ibid., p. 32.
30   H. Segal (1997) 'The uses and abuses of counter-transference', in Segal, *Psychoanalysis*, pp. 111–19.

10   Ronald Britton: Exclusions and Elegies

1   R. Britton (1998) *Belief and Imagination*, London: Routledge.
2   Biographical details are based on those kindly provided by Ronald Britton in 1998–9.
3   R. Britton (1997) 'Psychic reality and unconscious belief: A reply to Harold B. Gerard', *IJPA*, vol. 78, pp. 335–40.
4   R. Britton (1999) personal communication, 24 May.
5   R. Britton (1978) 'The deprived child', *The Practitioner: Journal of Postgraduate Medicine*, vol. 221, September, pp. 373–8.
6   R. Britton (1981) 'Re-enactment as an unwitting professional response to family dynamics', in S. Box et al., eds, *Psychotherapy with Families*, London: Routledge, pp. 48–58.
7   R. Britton (1983) 'Breakdown and reconstitution of the family circle', in M. Boston and R. Szur, eds, *Psychotherapy with Severely Deprived Children*, London: Maresfield, pp. 105–9.
8   S. Freud (1910) 'Contributions to the psychology of love I: A special type of choice of object made by men', *SE11*, pp. 165–75, 171.
9   R. Britton (1994) 'Publication anxiety', *IJPA*, vol. 75, pp. 1213–24.
10   R. Britton (1985) 'The Oedipus complex and the depressive position', *Sigmund Freud House Bulletin*, Vienna, vol. 9(1), pp. 7–12, revised (1992) as 'The Oedipus situation and the depressive position', in R. Anderson, ed., *Clinical Lectures on Klein and Bion*, London: Routledge, pp. 34–45.
11   Quoted by Britton in Anderson, ed., *Clinical Lectures*, p. 39.
12   Britton, in Anderson, ed., *Clinical Lectures*, p. 44.

13 R. Britton (1989) 'The missing link', in J. Steiner, ed., *The Oedipus Complex Today*, London: Karnac, pp. 83–101.
14 R. Britton (1992) 'Keeping things in mind', in Anderson, ed., *Clinical Lectures*, pp. 102–13 (113).
15 Marvell, 'Dialogue between the soul and the body', quoted by Britton, *Belief and Imegination*, p. 22.
16 R. Britton (1994) 'The blindness of the seeing eye', *Psychoanalytic Inquiry*, vol. 14(3), pp. 365–78.
17 R. Britton (1995) 'Psychic reality and unconscious belief', *IJPA*, vol. 76, pp. 19–23.
18 Quoted in Britton, *IJPA*, vol. 78, p. 338; see also G. Keynes (1967) *Blake*, London: Nonesuch, p. 139.
19 R. Britton (1999) 'Getting in on the act: The hysterical solution', *IJPA*, vol. 80(1), pp. 1–14.
20 Quoted in R. Britton (1997) 'The equilibrium between the paranoid-schizoid and depressive positions: Second thoughts', contribution to Bion Day conference, UCL, in Britton, *Belief and Imagination*, p. 132.
21 Britton, *Belief and Imagination*, p. 175.
22 Ibid.
23 Ibid., p. 169.
24 Ibid., p. 183.
25 Ibid., pp. 190–1.
26 Ibid., p. 192.
27 Ibid.
28 Ibid., p. 182.
29 Ibid., p. 117.
30 Ibid., pp. 129–30.
31 Ibid., p. 143.
32 Ibid., p. 130.
33 Ibid., p. 135.
34 Ibid., p. 155; Britton uses various translations of Rilke, in this case *The Selected Poetry of Rainer Maria Rilke*, ed. and trans. S. Mitchell (1987), London: Pan Books.
35 Ibid., p. 150.
36 Ibid., p. 151.
37 Ibid., p. 156.
38 Ibid.
39 Ibid., p. 157.
40 Ibid. For more on this topic, see R. Britton (1999) '"Primal grief" and "petrified rage": An exploration of Rilke's *Duino Elegies*', in D. Bell, ed., *Psychoanalysis and Culture*, London: Constable, pp. 27–47.
41 Britton, *Belief and Imagination*, p. 159.
42 Ibid.
43 Letter from Rilke to his Polish translator, November 1925, in J. B. Leishman (1936) 'Introduction', *Sonnets to Orpheus*, London: Hogarth, pp. 18–19. My thanks to Martin Golding for bringing to my attention Rilke's account in this letter of transforming what is outside into what is invisible within.

Index